D1357535

Ultrasound-Guided Regional Anesthesia in Children

A Practical Guide

Ultrasound-Guided Regional Anesthesia in Children

A Practical Guide

Edited by

Stephen Mannion
Consultant Anaesthetist, Department of Anaesthesiology, South Infirmary – Victoria University
Hospital, Cork and Senior Clinical Lecturer University College Cork, Ireland

Gabriella Iohom
Consultant Anaesthetist/Senior Lecturer, Department of Anaesthesia and Intensive Care Medicine,
Cork University Hospital and University College Cork, Cork, Ireland

Christophe Dadure
Professor of Anaesthesiology, Department of Anaesthesia and Critical Care Unit, Lapeyronie
University Hospital, Montpellier, France

Mark D. Reisbig
Assistant Professor of Anesthesiology in the Department of Anesthesiology, Creighton University
Medical Center, CHI Alegent Creighton Clinic, Omaha, NE, USA

Arjunan Ganesh
Associate Professor of Anesthesiology and Critical Care at the Hospital of the University of
Pennsylvania and the Children's Hospital of Philadelphia, Philadelphia, PA, USA

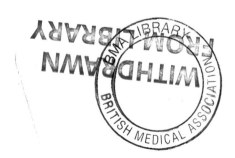
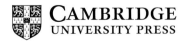
CAMBRIDGE
UNIVERSITY PRESS

CAMBRIDGE
UNIVERSITY PRESS

University Printing House, Cambridge CB2 8BS, United Kingdom

Cambridge University Press is part of the University of Cambridge.

It furthers the University's mission by disseminating knowledge
in the pursuit of education, learning and research at the highest
international levels of excellence.

www.cambridge.org
Information on this title: www.cambridge.org/9781107098770

© Cambridge University Press 2015

First published 2015

Printed in the United Kingdom by Bell and Bain Ltd

*A catalogue record for this publication is available from the British
Library*

Library of Congress Cataloguing in Publication data
Ultrasound-guided regional anesthesia in children : a practical guide /
edited by Stephen Mannion, Gabriella Iohom, Christophe Dadure,
Mark Reisbig, Arjunan Ganesh.
     p. ;   cm.
Includes bibliographical references and index.
ISBN 978-1-107-09877-0 (Hardback : alk. paper)
I. Mannion, Stephen, editor.   II. Iohom, Gabriella, editor.
III. Dadure, Christophe, editor.   IV. Reisbig, Mark, editor.
V. Ganesh, Arjunan, editor.
[DNLM: 1. Anesthesia, Conduction–methods.   2. Child.
3. Infant.   4. Intraoperative Complications–prevention & control.
5. Ultrasonography,
Interventional–methods. WO 300]
RD84
617.9′64083–dc23   2015006510

ISBN 978-1-107-09877-0 Hardback

Contents

v

Section 6 – Facial blocks

Contributors

Amr Abdelaal
Consultant Paediatric Anaesthetist, Addenbrookes Hospital, Cambridge, UK

Ahmed Abdel-Aziz
Consultant Paediatric Anaesthetist and Pediatric Intensivist, The James Cook University Hospital, Middlesborough, UK

Judith Barbaro-Brown
Teaching Fellow, Phase 1 Medicine, School for Medicine Pharmacy and Health, Durham University, Thornaby, Stockton-on-Tees, UK

Attila Bondár
Consultant Anaesthetist, Department of Anaesthesiology and Intensive Core Medicine, Semmelweis University, Budapest, Hungary

Christophe Dadure
Core Medicine Professor of Anesthesiology, Department of Anesthesia and Critical Care Unit, Lapeyronie University Hospital, Montpellier, France

Frédéric Duflo
Anesthesiologist, Department of Anesthesiology, Clinique du Val d'Ouest, Ecully, France

Éimhín Dunne
Clinical Fellow in Critical Care, King's College Hospital, London, UK

Arjunan Ganesh
Associate Professor of Anesthesiology and Critical Care, The Children's Hospital of Philadelphia and Perelman School of Medicine at University of Pennsylvania, Philadelphia, PA, USA

Anca Grigoras
Specialist in Anaesthesia, South Infirmary – Victoria University Hospital, Cork, Ireland

Harshad Gurnaney
Assistant Professor of Anesthesiology and Critical Care, The Children's Hospital of Philadelphia and Perelman School of Medicine at University of Pennsylvania, Philadelphia, PA, USA

Immanuel Hennessy
Specialist Registrar, Our Lady's Hospital for Sick Children, Crumlin, Dublin and South Infirmary – Victoria University Hospital, Cork, Ireland

Gabriella Iohom
Consultant Anaesthetist/Senior Lecturer, Department of Anaesthesia and Intensive Care Medicine, Cork University Hospital and University College Cork, Cork, Ireland

Peter Lee
Consultant Anaesthetist, Department of Anaesthesia, Intensive Care and Pain Medicine, Cork University Hospital, Cork, Ireland

Stephen Mannion
Consultant Anaesthetist, Department of Anaesthesiology, South Infirmary – Victoria University Hospital, Cork and Senior Clinical Lecturer, University College Cork, Ireland

Wallis T. Muhly
Assistant Professor of Anesthesiology and Critical Care, The Children's Hospital of Philadelphia and Perelman School of Medicine at University of Pennsylvania, Philadelphia, PA, USA

Jawad Mustafa
Consultant Anaesthetist, South Infirmary – Victoria University Hospital, Cork, Ireland

Brian O'Donnell
Consultant Anaesthetist BreastCheck and Cork University Hospital; Clinical Senior Lecturer ASSERT for Health Centre, University College Cork, Cork, Ireland

Pádraig O'Scanaill

Specialist Trainee in Anaesthesia, South Infirmary – Victoria University Hospital, Cork, Ireland

Mark D. Reisbig

Assistant Professor, Department of Anesthesiology, Creighton University School of Medicine; Consultant Anesthesiologist, Catholic Health Initiatives, Creighton University Medical Center, Omaha, NE, USA

Anne-Charlotte Saour

Consultant Anesthetist and Associate Professor, Department of Anesthesiology and Critical Care, Pediatric Anesthesia Unit, University Lapeyronie Hospital, Montpellier, France

Sinead O'Shaughnessy

Specialist Trainee in Anaesthesia, Department of Anaesthesiology, South Infirmary – Victoria University Hospital, Cork, Ireland

Chrystelle Sola

Consultant Anesthetist and Associate Professor, Department of Anesthesiology and Critical Care, Pediatric Anesthesia Unit, University Lapeyronie Hospital, Montpellier, France

Karthikeyan Kallidaikurichi Srinivasan

Specialist Registrar, Anaesthetics, Cork University Hospital, Cork, Ireland

Christina Van Horn

Assistant Professor, Department of Anesthesiology, Creighton University School of Medicine; Consultant Anesthesiologist, Catholic Health Initiatives, Creighton University Medical Center, Omaha, NE, USA

Charles Youngblood

Chairman and Assistant Professor, Department of Anesthesiology, Creighton University School of Medicine; Consultant Anesthesiologist, Catholic Health Initiatives, Creighton University Medical Center, Omaha, NE, USA

Introduction

Stephen Mannion

Introduction

Welcome to *Ultrasound-Guided Regional Anesthesia in Children*. If you are reading this book you will have both an interest in pediatrics and the use of regional anesthesia in caring for children.

Pediatric practice, regardless of its subspecialty status, is often viewed as the "Cinderella" of medicine, with innovations and clinical care usually following on from developments in adult practice.

A simple PubMed® search of the terms "children" and "regional anesthesia" reveals 227 results compared to 2069 for "regional anesthesia" on its own.[1] There is a lack of data upon which to base pediatric regional anesthesia practice and a substantial time lag behind changes that occur in adult practice.

Bernard Dalens attempted to address some of these knowledge deficits in his reference textbook *Pediatric Regional Anesthesia*, the first edition of which was released in 1989 (Dalens, 1989). Currently there is a lack of books available on regional anesthesia in children. The majority of anesthesiologists have to refer to general regional anesthesia resources where pediatric regional anesthesia is represented only by a subsection.

Benefits

Anesthesiologists specializing in pediatrics are well aware of the benefits that regional anesthesia techniques bring to the care of children (Russell et al., 2013). The main benefits of regional anesthesia in children are improved post-operative analgesia and a reduction in the use of opioids, with a concomitant

Table 1.1 Benefits of regional anesthesia in children

Reduced pain scores
Reduced opioid consumption
Decreased post-operative nausea and vomiting (PONV)
Reduced minimum alveolar concentration
Reduced use of muscle relaxants
Reduced emergence delirium
Greater hemodynamic stability
Reduced immunosuppression
Greater suppression of metabolic response
Less post-operative respiratory support after major surgery
Earlier return of gut function and feeding
Reduced intensive care unit stay
Shorter hospital stay

reduction in associated adverse effects, such as nausea and vomiting, excessive sedation, and respiratory compromise (Bosenberg, 2013) (Table 1.1).

Recent concerns regarding the possible adverse effects of drugs used in general anesthesia on neurodevelopment, and in particular on cognitive and behavioral outcomes in later life, have prompted discussion of the benefits of regional anesthesia techniques as the sole anesthetic for children undergoing surgery (Lei et al., 2014).

The use of regional anesthesia in perioperative care and as part of the management of pain in children is common, with peripheral nerve blocks now accounting for two-thirds of all neural blocks performed as compared to 20 years ago when they made up just one-third (Ecoffey et al., 2010).

---

[1] PubMed® search results. Available at http://www.ncbi.nlm.nih.gov/pubmed/?term=children+%22regional+anaesthesia%22 (Accessed October 21, 2014).

Ultrasound-Guided Regional Anesthesia in Children, ed. Mannion et al. Published by Cambridge University Press.
© Cambridge University Press 2015.

Challenges

The practice of regional anesthesia in children is not without its challenges.

Unlike in adults, in the vast majority of children (95%), regional anesthesia is performed with the child under general anesthesia (Polaner et al., 2012). This practice appears to be safe in children and may well be unavoidable in many children so as to prevent movement.

Success rates of neural blockade in children are often difficult to determine because of the concurrent use of general anesthesia, as well as the difficulties in eliciting specific information on sensory or motor blockade in young children. Traditional landmark-based techniques have variable success rates, even when combined with nerve stimulation (Ponde and Diwan, 2009).

These factors mean that it is important to ensure reliable, high rates of successful neural blockade if we are considering regional anesthesia in children.

One of the major concerns in caring for children is safety. There are unique elements in performing regional anesthesia in children compared to adults. Children are not a heterogeneous group and present at a wide range of ages, from preterm babies to 15-year-old adolescents. These various ages present a spectrum of physiologic, anatomic, and pharmacologic parameters relevant to the practice of regional anesthesia (Steward and Lerman, 2001).

Small differences in local anesthetic (LA) dosage or volume injected may have significant adverse effects. Regional anesthetic techniques that would allow for a reduction in both, should, therefore, offer a safer method.

Ultrasound

The use of ultrasonography in regional anesthesia is a recent development. In South Africa, la Grange and colleagues described the first use of Doppler ultrasound to perform a supraclavicular block (la Grange et al., 1978). It took until 1994 for what might be considered the routine practice of ultrasound for regional anesthesia – that is the use of ultrasound to view the nerve, needle, and LA – to be first published by Kapral and colleagues (Kapral et al., 1994). Ten years later the same group published the first randomized trial of the use of ultrasound to perform regional anesthesia in children (Marhofer et al., 2004), which followed on from a case report a year earlier on ultrasound-guided sciatic nerve block (Gray et al., 2003).

The use of ultrasound has revolutionized the practice of regional anesthesia, as demonstrated by year-on-year increases in the number of publications in the field (Figure 1.1). This "ultrasound revolution" includes the performance of regional anesthesia in children (Boretsky, 2014).

Many of the challenges associated with the performance of regional anesthesia in children may be significantly ameliorated by the application of ultrasound, due to visualization of critical structures, reduced LA volumes, improved success rates, and reduced rate of vascular puncture.

Need

This book addresses the need to encourage the use, and improve the performance, of regional anesthesia using ultrasound in children.

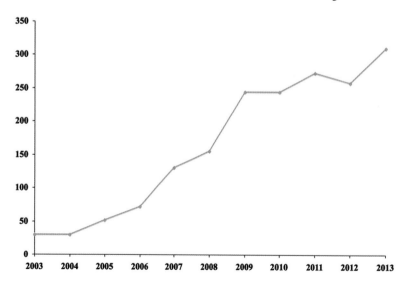

Figure 1.1 Graph of PubMed® search results for terms "ultrasound," "nerve," and "block" from 2003 to 2013.

There are few resources available, either in print and online, that specifically focus on the use of ultrasound in pediatric regional anesthesia practice.

This book has been conceived with the practicing anesthesiologist in mind. The editors determined that a practical, user-friendly book would be an excellent tool to encourage and improve the use of ultrasound in pediatric regional anesthesia. They have assembled an international group of authors who have written this up-to-date guide on specific ultrasound-guided blocks.

Other users, such as emergency doctors, pain specialists, nurse anesthetists, and medical students, may also find this book useful.

Practical

This book consists of two parts. The first part contains five chapters dedicated to the principles and practice of ultrasound use for regional anesthesia in children.

These chapters address in detail the challenges and issues described previously and include the performance of regional anesthesia in children, the pharmacology of LAs in children, the "nuts and bolts" of ultrasonography, managing safety and complications, and providing a description of the relevant clinical anatomy to allow interpretation of the sonoanatomy for each nerve block. These chapters should be read before performing any block, as the principles and practices necessary for safe regional anesthesia in children are described in detail and are not repeated in the "block" chapters.

The second part consists of 15 chapters, each describing the performance of a nerve block using ultrasound. Each "block" chapter will introduce the nerve block and describe its clinical uses and the current literature on the use of ultrasound for that block. The chapter will provide a practical "how-to-do" section on performing that block, including relevant sonoanatomy, patient and probe position, needle placement, and block performance. The reader should note that static ultrasound images are not fully representative of scanning in practice. The dynamic imaging obtained by subtle tilting and translation of the probe results in better resolution images in real-time. Therefore, the sonoanatomy has been labeled to assist with anatomic identification, and where necessary for quality purposes, a needle pathway has been highlighted as for some blocks the needle images were faint, poor, or unclear. Finally a section on clinical tips is provided, where applicable, from the clinical experiences of the authors.

Each chapter has a suggested reading list including references from the text as well as resources that provide further information for interested readers.

Some readers may be disappointed by the apparent omission of certain nerve blocks. Examples of techniques where ultrasound guidance can be used include penile and psoas compartment blocks. The non-inclusion of a particular block does not diminish its clinical usefulness; we have chosen the nerve blocks for this book based on their clinical application, common usage, and/or innovative nature.

Conclusion

The safe and effective practice of regional anesthesia in children requires in-depth knowledge and supervised training. This book in isolation will not make you an expert in pediatric ultrasound-guided regional anesthesia. It will, we hope, assist you in developing and expanding your skills and knowledge base and facilitate the application of regional anesthesia to your everyday pediatric practice.

Acknowledgements

I would like to thank my co-editors for their commitment and enthusiasm and Dr. Peter Lee who has been a regular sounding board, his insights and comments on this project were very welcome. I want to thank Kristina Mannion for her photography work on the patient and probe position images. Finally I want to thank four of my other children; Isabelle, Zoë, Ella, and Adam Mannion for their time and patience in their role as models for most of the blocks in this book.

Suggested reading

Boretsky KR. (2014) Regional anesthesia in pediatrics: marching forward. *Curr Opin Anaesthesiol.* 27,556–60.

Bosenberg AT. (2013) Regional anaesthesia in children: an update. *South Afr J Anaesth Analg.* 19,282–8.

Dalens BJ. (1989). *Pediatric Regional Anesthesia.* Boca Raton, FL: CRC Press.

Ecoffey C, Lacroix F, Giaufré E, Orliaguet G, Courrèges P; Association des Anesthésistes Réanimateurs Pédiatriques d'Expression Française (ADARPEF). (2010) Epidemiology and morbidity of regional anesthesia in children: a follow-up one-year prospective survey of the

French-Language Society of Paediatric Anaesthesiologists (ADARPEF). *Paediatr Anaesth.* 20,1061–9.

Gray AT, Collins AB, Schafhalter-Zoppoth I. (2003) Sciatic nerve block in a child: a sonographic approach. *Anesth Analg.* 97, 1300–2.

Kapral S, Krafft P, Eibenberger K, et al. (1994) Ultrasound-guided supraclavicular approach for regional anesthesia of the brachial plexus. *Anesth Analg.* 78, 507–13.

Kim HS, Kim CS, Kim SD, Lee JR. (2011) Fascia iliaca compartment block reduces emergence agitation by providing effective analgesic properties in children. *J Clin Anesth.* 23,119–23.

la Grange P, Foster PA, Pretorius LK. (1978) Application of the Doppler ultrasound bloodflow detector in supraclavicular brachial plexus block. *Br J Anaesth.* 50,965–7.

Lei SY, Hache M, Loepke AW. (2014) Clinical research into anesthetic neurotoxicity: does anesthesia cause neurological abnormalities in humans? *J Neurosurg Anesthesiol.* 26,349–57.

Marhofer P, Sitzwohl C, Greher M, Kapral S. (2004) Ultrasound guidance for infraclavicular brachial plexus anaesthesia in children. *Anaesthesia.* 59,642–6.

Polaner DM, Taenzer AH, Walker BJ, et al. (2012). Pediatric Regional Anesthesia Network (PRAN): a multi-institutional study of the use and incidence of complications of pediatric regional anesthesia. *Anesth Analg.* 115,1353–64.

Ponde VC, Diwan S. (2009) Does ultrasound guidance improve the success rate of infraclavicular brachial plexus block when compared with nerve stimulation in children with radial club hands? *Anesth Analg.* 108,1967–70.

Russell P, von Ungern-Sternberg BS, Schug SA. (2013). Perioperative analgesia in pediatric surgery. *Curr Opin Anaesthesiol.* 26,420–7.

Sinha A, Sood J. (2012) Caudal block and emergence delirium in pediatric patients: is it analgesia or sedation? *Saudi J Anaesth.* 6,403–7.

Steward DJ, Lerman J. (2001). *Manual of Pediatric Anesthesia.* Philadelphia, PA: Churchill Livingstone.

Chapter

2

Performance of regional anesthesia in children

Arjunan Ganesh and Wallis T. Muhly

Introduction

The use of regional anesthesia for post-operative analgesia in children has gained popularity over time. While the caudal block is still the most commonly performed regional anesthetic technique in children, the performance of peripheral nerve blocks is growing. Advances in ultrasound technology have certainly contributed to the increase in the use of regional anesthetic techniques in children. The ability to view the anatomy and the use of real-time needle guidance has increased the confidence among anesthesiologists to perform a variety of regional anesthetic procedures in anesthetized children.

A successful regional anesthetic block requires adequate distribution of local anesthetic (LA) around the target neural structures (Marhofer et al., 2005). The ability to visualize the spread of LA adjacent to the neural structures has improved the success of regional anesthetic techniques. In addition, variations in anatomy can be recognized with the use of ultrasound, which in turn has the potential to increase the safety and success of regional anesthetic techniques.

This chapter describes the key principles necessary for performing safe and effective ultrasound-guided regional anesthesia in children – a number of the topics are considerably expanded on in subsequent chapters.

Anatomy and physiology

Chapter 6 describes the relevant anatomy for the blocks described in this book – below is a brief outline of the key anatomic differences between children and adults.

With regard to peripheral nerve blocks anatomic differences between children and adults may not be significant, although the smaller size of infants and children (structures are more superficial compared to adults) allow the use of higher frequency ultrasound probes resulting in a higher resolution image. However, one needs to appreciate the differences with neuraxial blockade. In a study using ultrasound guidance for epidural placement in children, the median value for the termination of the spinal cord was noted to be L2, but was as low as L3/L4 in some neonates (Willschke et al., 2007). Also, the dural sac in infants extends up to the S3 level. This is in contrast to adults where the spinal cord ends at the level of L1 and the dural sac at S1. Practitioners need to keep this in mind when performing neuraxial blockade in order to avoid injury to the spinal cord or an unintentional intrathecal injection. However, in infants under six months old, the posterior elements of the spinal canal are incompletely ossified allowing an acoustic window for sonographic imaging. With increasing age, the value of ultrasound imaging decreases as ossification increases and the depth of the epidural space and spinal cord increases (Willschke et al., 2006). The authors in this study also determined the paramedian longitudinal and the intervertebral axial planes offer the best views, but the size of these ultrasound windows also decreases with age.

Spinal anesthesia, more commonly used as the sole anesthetic technique in neonates for procedures below the T10 level, may reduce the incidence of post-operative apnea in this population. Larger doses of LA are needed in infants for reasons that include larger cerebrospinal fluid (CSF) volume in relation to body weight (4 ml/kg vs. 2 ml/kg in adults), greater height-to-body weight ratio in infants and a larger surface area of the spinal cord. It is also rare to see profound hypotension with spinal anesthesia in infants and young children (Dohi et al., 1979; Dohi and Seino, 1986), which could be due to an immature sympathetic nervous system and smaller blood volume in the lower extremities of a small child.

Ultrasound-Guided Regional Anesthesia in Children, ed. Mannion et al. Published by Cambridge University Press.
© Cambridge University Press 2015.

Regional anesthesia under general anesthesia

The decision to perform regional anesthesia in anesthetized or heavily sedated patients is controversial and made in the absence of reliable scientific evidence (Bernards et al., 2008). In this article, the authors have acknowledged that when awake, infants and young children may be unable to communicate symptoms of potential nerve injury or intravascular injection of LA, and also uncontrolled movement in this age group may increase the risk of injury. Therefore, they have recommended that performance of neuraxial and peripheral nerve blocks in anesthetized or heavily sedated children may be carried out when benefits outweigh the risks. However, reports of permanent spinal cord injury in four patients in whom interscalene blocks were placed under general anesthesia (Benumof, 2000) had prompted the authors (Bernards et al., 2008) to recommend against performing interscalene blocks under general anesthesia in children.

Several prospective databases have attempted to define the additional risk, if any, when regional anesthesia is performed under general anesthesia in children (Giaufre et al., 1996; Polaner et al., 2012; Taenzer et al., 2014a, 2014b). In their study (Polaner et al., 2012), the authors reported that 95% of regional anesthetic procedures in children were performed under general anesthesia with a very low rate of complications. Two years later (Taenzer et al., 2014b), using additional information from the database, the authors concluded that performance of regional anesthetic procedures under general anesthesia did not increase the risk of complications when compared to procedures performed in awake/sedated children. In fact, the authors noticed a tendency towards a lower rate of complications when regional anesthesia was performed under general anesthesia. However, there were limitations to this study including a lack of a matched comparison based on age groups and blocks. Another recent study from the Pediatric Regional Anesthesia Network (PRAN) group (Taenzer et al., 2014a) evaluated the safety of interscalene blocks in children and adolescents under general anesthesia. They concluded that placement of interscalene blocks under general anesthesia in children is no less safe than placement in awake adults as far as post-operative neurologic symptoms or LA systemic toxicity (LAST), and questioned the American Society of Regional Anesthesia and Pain Medicine (ASRA) advisory against performing interscalene blocks under general anesthesia in pediatric patients.

The use of ultrasound guidance for peripheral nerve blocks may help improve the safety of procedures performed under general anesthesia. The ability to localize the tip of the needle and monitor the spread of LA along with advances in ultrasound technology may improve the safety of peripheral nerve blocks, particularly the interscalene block.

The present consensus among almost all pediatric regional anesthesia enthusiasts is that it is safe to perform peripheral nerve and neuraxial blockade under general anesthesia, which is based primarily on large case series (Giaufre et al., 1996; Krane et al., 1998; Llewellyn and Moriarty, 2007; Berde and Greco, 2012; Polaner et al., 2012).

Pharmacology

In most cases, pediatric regional anesthesia is performed as an adjunct to general anesthesia during the intraoperative period and primarily for postoperative analgesia. As such, lower concentrations of LA can be used in pediatric peripheral nerve blockade. Ropivacaine is more popular than bupivacaine both for bolus injections in all patients, and particularly in infants for epidural infusions (Feldman et al., 1989; Dony et al., 2000; Bosenberg et al., 2005). Several adjuvants including clonidine, opioids, dexamethasone, epinephrine, dexmedetomidine, and others have been used with varying results. The use of ultrasound can decrease the minimal effective volume of LA required (Marhofer et al., 1998; Casati et al., 2007), and could, thus, increase safety. Finally, the immediate availability of Intralipid®, when performing regional anesthetic procedures, has become a standard of care (Weinberg, 2010; Neal et al., 2012). Please refer to Chapters 3 and 4 for detailed description of pharmacology and management of LA toxicity.

Informed consent

Consent requires five conditions to make it acceptable: (1) the patient must be competent; (2) information must be disclosed; (3) the patient must understand the information; (4) the consent must be voluntary; and (5) the patient gives authorization (Ecoffey and Dalens, 2003). The issue of competency, which is better defined in adults, is still quite complicated in children. In most countries, a child is considered to be an adult at the age of 18 years, although some jurisdictions allow children 16 years and older to consent to a medical or dental procedure.

However, in children who have attained a certain level of maturity and are able to make reasonable choices regarding their care, it may be prudent to respect their wishes. This may particularly be true when regional anesthesia is considered as part of the anesthetic plan. As an example, there are children who, because of previous experience, may refuse continuous epidural analgesia because of the need to maintain an indwelling Foley catheter while the epidural catheter is in place. There may be children or adolescents who choose to forgo continuous perineural infusion techniques because of being uncomfortable with the concept of being attached to nerve catheters and infusion devices. Interestingly, we have even encountered patients who did not like the feeling of a numb extremity and requested premature removal of their perineural catheter. Enthusiastic anesthesiologists need to respect the wishes of children and parents who refuse any form of regional anesthesia, even when they believe that it will offer superior pain relief, as other analgesic alternatives may be adequate and more acceptable to the family.

There is an increasing drive and directive by federal agencies to increase the participation of children in research. The informed consent process for research in children usually involves proxy consent from the parents and obtaining assent from the children who attain a certain age and maturity. The criteria for obtaining assent vary from one institution to another. Because children and adolescents will increasingly be recruited to be research subjects, it is imperative that investigators better understand, from both the child's and parents' perspective, (1) how decisions are made about research enrolment, and (2) how current practices of informed consent/assent can be improved to foster respect for children and to protect child subjects from research risks (Broome et al., 2003).

Use of ultrasound

The use of ultrasound for peripheral nerve blocks will soon become the gold standard for peripheral nerve blocks. Several studies have shown the benefits of ultrasound guidance that includes faster onset time, higher success rate, and decreased minimal effective volume (Marhofer et al., 1998; Casati et al., 2007).

Ultrasound guidance should be a clear choice in performance of blocks involving fascial planes, namely transversus abdominis plane, ilioinguinal (Willschke et al., 2005), and rectus sheath blocks, where the other alternative is to rely on pops and clicks (Griffin and Nicholls, 2010). However, there is a learning curve involved in the use of ultrasound. Although many anesthesiology training programs offer training in performance of ultrasound-guided blocks, the experience is not uniform. Also, very few programs offer a structured training program in the use of ultrasound guidance. Despite these issues, the use of ultrasound guidance is increasing in clinical practice as the technology is improving and the costs are decreasing. In the PRAN study (Polaner et al., 2012), about 82% of upper extremity, 70% of lower extremity, and most truncal blocks were performed with ultrasound guidance. The use of ultrasound for neuraxial blockade, though reported (Willschke et al., 2006, 2007), requires further study before broad recommendations can be made.

The cost of an ultrasound machine is often a hurdle in acquiring this technology in various departments. In a study comparing infraclavicular block using nerve stimulator and ultrasound guidance, it was demonstrated that it was cost efficient with ultrasound guidance (Sandhu et al., 2004). In addition, ultrasound guidance is also increasingly being used for central line placement, arterial line placement, and in cases of difficult intravenous access. Please refer to Chapter 5 for a thorough discussion of the use of ultrasound in pediatric regional anesthesia.

Equipment

The primary equipment in ultrasound-guided regional anesthesia is the ultrasound machine. The selection of machine in each institution may be determined by the practitioners' personal preferences, features in the machine, cost, and institutional contracts with manufacturers who provide other devices (Figure 2.1). However, the following capabilities are recommended: (1) easy to use, in order for practitioners of varying abilities to use; (2) portable; (3) a selection of linear, curvilinear, and phased array probes; (4) color-flow Doppler; (5) image- and video-capture facilities for documentation and training; and (6) a suitable warranty (Griffin and Nicholls, 2010).

A variety of needles, stimulating and non-stimulating, and echogenic needles that are coated or scored are available for use (Figure 2.2). In centers where only ultrasound guidance is used, stimulating needles are not necessary. However, many practitioners still use a combination of nerve stimulation and ultrasound guidance. There also are echogenic catheters available for placement. At this moment there is no clear evidence to show the benefit of echogenic needles and catheters. A variety of nerve stimulators are available if one uses a concurrent nerve stimulation technique.

Long-sleeve probe covers are recommended when perineural catheters are placed. For single injection blocks one can just seal the probe tips with sterile adhesives (Figure 2.3).

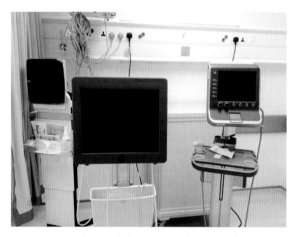

Figure 2.1 A selection of ultrasound machines used for regional anesthesia.

Block set up

All patients should have the standard monitors that include pulse oximetry, electrocardiogram (ECG), and blood pressure in addition to a functioning intravenous (IV) line prior to the placement of a block. As most regional anesthetic procedures in children are performed under general anesthesia, one should remember to avoid neuromuscular blockade if nerve stimulation is to be used for performance of the block. The ability to use neuromuscular blockade is an advantage when performing blocks with ultrasound guidance only. Also, when performing the blocks under general anesthesia, there should be assistance available to monitor the patient. The second person may also help with optimizing the ultrasound image, operating the nerve stimulator when used, and injection of the LA. It is also important to pay attention to ergonomics, like raising the table to the desired height and lining up the ultrasound machine, the needle direction, and the line of vision to obtain best results.

Drugs needed for resuscitation, such as epinephrine and Intralipid®, should be readily available to address LAST if it occurs. When blocks are performed in awake/sedated patients, equipment for airway support should be available along with benzodiazepines to treat seizures.

Asepsis

Recent guidelines on the prevention of regional anesthesia-related infection have recommended the

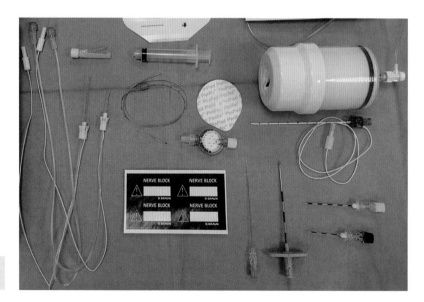

Figure 2.2 A variety of needles can be used for ultrasound-guided regional anesthesia. A nerve stimulator can be used concurrently with many block needles if required. A catheter should be labeled with a suitable label, e.g. "nerve block," and can be connected with an elastomeric pump such as the one shown. Needles shown from left to right are: 50 mm and 25 mm 21-gauge stimulating needles; 27-gauge spinal pencil point needle (orange); 18-gauge Touhy-type needle (blue); 20-gauge Touhy-type catheter through needle (green); and pediatric caudal needles – 20-gauge (yellow) and 22-gauge (black).

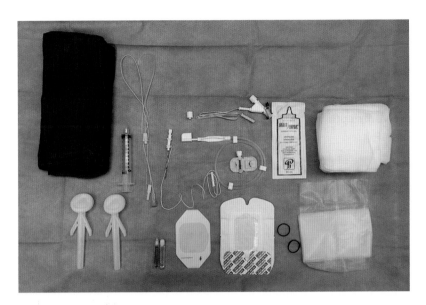

Figure 2.3 Sterile set-up for an ultrasound-guided peripheral nerve block with catheter placement – includes sterile skin disinfectant, drape, sterile gel and probe cover, and catheter skin adhesive and clear dressing.

use of chlorhexidine in alcohol solutions for all blocks including neuraxial (ASRA 2006; ASA 2010; AAGBI 2014). However, there is ongoing controversy in this area, which is beyond the scope of this chapter. In summary, skin preparation for peripheral nerve blocks can be done using either iodine or chlorhexidine solutions mixed with alcohol. In the case of neuraxial blocks, concerns that chlorhexidine is a neural toxic and that it has been implicated in cases of chemical arachnoiditis in adults have resulted in vigorous debate regarding its use for neuraxial blocks. The most recently published national guidelines (UK and Ireland) recommend chlorhexidine in 70% isopropyl alcohol but at a reduced concentration of 0.5%.

When perineural catheters are placed it is advisable to drape the field just like for a surgical procedure (Figure 2.3). The incidence of infection following placement of perineural catheters in children is less than 1% (Ganesh et al., 2007; Polaner et al., 2012; Gurnaney et al., 2014) and for neuraxial blockade, about 1.1% (Polaner et al., 2012) and less than 1% (Llewellyn and Moriarty, 2007). In most studies there was a clear correlation between the duration of the indwelling catheter and the risk of infection. The incidence of serious infective complications like epidural abscess and meningitis was very low.

Safety and complications

The safety of regional anesthesia in children has been well established (Giaufre et al., 1996; Krane et al.,

1998; Llewellyn and Moriarty, 2007; Polaner et al., 2012; Krane and Polaner, 2014; Taenzer et al., 2014b). The incidence of neurologic complications is extremely low and infective complications are mostly confined to local skin infections. There were no cases of deep-seated abscesses in the PRAN study (Polaner et al., 2012) and only 2 cases (out of 10 633 epidurals) in the Pediatric Epidural Audit (Llewellyn and Moriarty, 2007).

A prospective study of 1010 ultrasound-guided blocks found neurologic symptoms in 8.2% of patients after 10 days, 3.7% after 1 month, and 0.6% after 6 months (Fredrickson and Kilfoyle, 2009), which is similar to the overall incidence of complications following peripheral nerve blocks (Auroy et al., 2002). Chapter 4 deals with complications in greater detail. There are no large pediatric studies to evaluate the safety of ultrasound-guided regional anesthesia in children. The incidence of adverse events following peripheral nerve blockade is so low that it is going to be very difficult to demonstrate a superior safety profile with the use of ultrasound guidance. However, the improved success rate and the requirement for lower volumes with the use of ultrasound guidance should result in the increasing use of ultrasound for peripheral nerve blockade.

Interestingly, there has been renewed interest in regional anesthesia as the sole anesthetic technique in children. The effects of general anesthesia drugs on neurodevelopment, particularly on behavioral and cognitive function, has recently added to this debate

(Lei et al. 2014). Spinal anesthesia previously performed in neonates or for children at increased risk of apnea, can be safely and effectively performed in older children as well. A pediatric series of 1132 spinal anesthetics for lower abdominal and orthopedic surgeries, in children aged 6 months to 14 years, has been published without a major complication (Puncuh et al. 2004).

Contraindications to regional anesthesia

Contraindications to regional anesthesia in children are very similar to those in adults. Parent or patient refusal, infection at the site, and LA allergy are absolute contraindications. Coagulopathy due to disorders of coagulation, use of anticoagulants, and systemic disorders like overt sepsis are usually absolute contraindications for neuraxial blockade. However, peripheral nerve blockade may be performed with caution in some of these patients (Sripada et al., 2009), but they should be closely monitored for complications with early intervention when indicated (Rodriguez et al., 2011). Imaging with ultrasound prior to neuraxial procedures in infants, particularly those with atypical dimples that are large (>5 mm), high on the back (>2.5 cm from the anus), or appear in combination with other lesions (that include hemangiomas, hairy patches, etc.), may help detect cases of spinal dysraphism and thereby prevent catastrophic consequences (Kriss and Desai, 1998). Relative contraindications include progressive neurologic diseases and the presence of ventriculo-peritoneal shunts (Ecoffey, 2012).

Post-operative care

Whenever feasible all patients who have had a regional anesthetic procedure performed in the operating room need to be evaluated in the recovery room to evaluate the efficacy of the block. This is important as most regional anesthetic techniques in children are performed under general anesthesia and success of the block can only be truly determined in the postoperative period. Supplement analgesia should be ordered for those who have insufficient coverage from the block or when the block is a failure. Pain assessment should be carried out in the recovery room and at least every 4 hours thereafter. Clear instructions need to be given to protect the insensate areas resulting from the block. If there is a possibility of motor blockade, particularly in the lower extremities, adequate weight-bearing instructions need to be provided. In case of continuous peripheral nerve and neuraxial blockade, the catheter site needs to be evaluated at least once a day to look for signs of infection/dislodgement.

When patients are discharged home with indwelling perineural catheters, verbal and written education should be provided about the continuous infusion device system, techniques to remove the catheter, recognition of potential complications (symptoms of LA systemic toxicity), catheter dislodgement, and inadequate pain control. Families should also receive emergency contact information for the pain service. Patients should be cautioned to avoid weight bearing on the extremities that are weak and also to protect insensate areas from injury (e.g. from heat, cold, pressure, and other trauma) (Ganesh et al., 2007; Gurnaney et al., 2014).

Conclusions

Regional anesthesia in children is gaining in popularity. The availability of safety data from several multi-center prospective and retrospective studies has helped pediatric anesthesiologists approach regional anesthesia with renewed interest. The advances in ultrasound technology and its availability have accelerated this resurgence. More data should be available in the future to understand the full impact of the use of ultrasound guidance in pediatric regional anesthesia.

Suggested reading

Auroy Y, Benhamou D, Bargues L., et al. (2002) Major complications of regional anesthesia in France: the SOS Regional Anesthesia Hotline Service. *Anesthesiology.* 97,1274–80.

Benumof JL. (2000) Permanent loss of cervical spinal cord function associated with interscalene block performed under general anesthesia. *Anesthesiology.* 93,1541–4.

Berde C, Greco C. (2012) Pediatric regional anesthesia: drawing inferences on safety from prospective registries and case reports. *Anesth Analg.* 115, 1259–62.

Bernards CM, Hadzic A, Suresh S, Neal JM. (2008) Regional anesthesia in anesthetized or heavily sedated patients. *Reg Anesth Pain Med.* 33,449–60.

Bosenberg AT, Thomas J, Cronje L, et al. (2005) Pharmacokinetics and efficacy of ropivacaine for continuous epidural infusion in neonates and infants. *Paediatr Anaesth.* 15,739–49.

Broome ME, Kodish E, Geller G, Siminoff LA. (2003) Children in research: new perspectives and practices for informed consent. *IRB.* Suppl 25(5),S20–3.

Casati A, Baciarello M, Di Cianni S, et al. (2007) Effects of ultrasound guidance on the minimum effective anaesthetic volume required to block the femoral nerve. *Br J Anaesth.* 98,823–7.

Dohi S, Seino H. (1986). Spinal anesthesia in premature infants: dosage and effects of sympathectomy. *Anesthesiology.* 65,559–61.

Dohi S, Naito H, Takahashi T. (1979) Age-related changes in blood pressure and duration of motor block in spinal anesthesia. *Anesthesiology.* 50,319–23.

Dony P, Dewinde V, Vanderick B, et al. (2000). The comparative toxicity of ropivacaine and bupivacaine at equipotent doses in rats. *Anesth Analg.* 91,1489–92.

Ecoffey C. (2012) Safety in pediatric regional anesthesia. *Paediatr Anaesth.* 22,25–30.

Ecoffey C, Dalens B. (2003). Informed consent for children. *Curr Opin Anaesthesiol.* 16,205–8.

Feldman HS, Arthur GR, Covino BG. (1989) Comparative systemic toxicity of convulsant and supraconvulsant doses of intravenous ropivacaine, bupivacaine, and lidocaine in the conscious dog. *Anesth Analg.* 69,794–801.

Fredrickson MJ, Kilfoyle DH. (2009) Neurological complication analysis of 1000 ultrasound guided peripheral nerve blocks for elective orthopaedic surgery: a prospective study. *Anaesthesia.* 64,836–44.

Ganesh A, Rose JB, Wells L, et al. (2007) Continuous peripheral nerve blockade for inpatient and outpatient postoperative analgesia

in children. *Anesth Analg.* 105,1234–42.

Giaufre E, Dalens B, Gombert A. (1996). Epidemiology and morbidity of regional anesthesia in children: a one-year prospective survey of the French-Language Society of Pediatric Anesthesiologists. *Anesth Analg.* 83,904–12.

Griffin J, Nicholls B. (2010) Ultrasound in regional anaesthesia. *Anaesthesia.* 65 (Suppl 1),1–12.

Gurnaney H, Kraemer FW, Maxwell L, et al. (2014) Ambulatory continuous peripheral nerve blocks in children and adolescents: a longitudinal 8-year single center study. *Anesth Analg.* 118,621–7.

Krane EJ, Polaner D. (2014) The safety and effectiveness of continuous peripheral nerve blockade in children. *Anesth Analg.* 118, 499–500.

Krane EJ, Dalens BJ, Murat I, Murrell D. (1998) The safety of epidurals placed during general anesthesia. *Reg Anesth Pain Med.* 23,433–8.

Kriss VM, Desai NS. (1998) Occult spinal dysraphism in neonates: assessment of high-risk cutaneous stigmata on sonography. *AJR Am J Roentgenol.* 171,1687–92.

Lei SY, Hache M, Loepke AW. (2014). Clinical research into anesthetic neurotoxicity: does anesthesia cause neurological abnormalities in humans? *J Neurosurg Anesthesiol.* 26,349–57.

Llewellyn N, Moriarty A. (2007). The national pediatric epidural audit. *Paediatr Anaesth.* 17,520–33.

Marhofer P, Schrogendorfer K, Wallner T, et al. (1998). Ultrasonographic guidance reduces the amount of local anesthetic for 3-in-1 blocks. *Reg Anesth Pain Med.* 23,584–8.

Marhofer P, Greher M, Kapral S. (2005). Ultrasound guidance in regional anaesthesia. *Br J Anaesth.* 94,7–17.

Neal JM, Bernards CM, Butterworth JFT, et al. (2010) ASRA practice advisory on local anesthetic systemic toxicity. *Reg Anesth Pain Med.* 35,152–61.

Neal JM, Mulroy MF, Weinberg GL. (2012) American Society of Regional Anesthesia and Pain Medicine checklist for managing local anesthetic systemic toxicity: 2012 version. *Reg Anesth Pain Med.* 37,16–18.

Polaner DM, Taenzer AH, Walker BJ, et al. (2012) Pediatric Regional Anesthesia Network (PRAN): a multi-institutional study of the use and incidence of complications of pediatric regional anesthesia. *Anesth Analg.* 115,1353–64.

Puncuh F, Lampugnani E, Kokki H. (2004) Use of spinal anaesthesia in paediatric patients: a single centre experience with 1132 cases. *Paediatr Anaesth.* 14,564–7.

Rodriguez J, Taboada M, Garcia F, et al. (2011) Intraneural hematoma after nerve stimulation-guided femoral block in a patient with factor XI deficiency: case report. *J Clin Anesth.* 23,234–7.

Sandhu NS, Sidhu DS, Capan LM. (2004) The cost comparison of infraclavicular brachial plexus block by nerve stimulator and ultrasound guidance. *Anesth Analg.* 98,267–8.

Sripada R, Reyes JJ, Sun R. (2009) Peripheral nerve blocks for intraoperative management in patients with hemophilia A. *J Clin Anesth.* 21,120–3.

Taenzer AH, Walker BJ, Bosenberg AT, et al. (2014a) Interscalene brachial plexus blocks under general anesthesia in children: is this safe practice? A report from the Pediatric Regional Anesthesia Network (PRAN). *Reg Anesth Pain Med.* 39,502–5.

Taenzer AH, Walker BJ, Bosenberg AT, et al. (2014b). Asleep versus awake: does it matter? Pediatric regional block complications by patient state: a report from the Pediatric Regional Anesthesia

Network. *Reg Anesth Pain Med.* 39,279–83.

Weinberg GL. (2010) Treatment of local anesthetic systemic toxicity (LAST). *Reg Anesth Pain Med.* 35,188–93.

Willschke H, Marhofer P, Bosenberg A, et al. (2005) Ultrasonography for ilioinguinal/iliohypogastric nerve blocks in children. *Br J Anaesth.* 95,226–30.

Willschke H, Marhofer P, Bosenberg A, et al. (2006) Epidural catheter placement in children: comparing a novel approach using ultrasound guidance and a standard loss-of-resistance technique. *Br J Anaesth.* 97,200–7.

Willschke H, Bosenberg A, Marhofer P, et al. (2007) Epidural catheter placement in neonates: sonoanatomy and feasibility of ultrasonographic guidance in term and preterm neonates. *Reg Anesth Pain Med.* 32,34–40.

Chapter

3

Pharmacology of local anesthetics in children

Christina Van Horn and Mark D. Reisbig

Introduction

Regional anesthesia has been shown to have a number of benefits including a reduction in stress response and inflammation, reduced opioid consumption and related side effects, and better post-operative analgesia (Roberts, 2006).

The use of local anesthetic (LA) is a prerequisite for successful nerve blockade; however, adverse outcomes such as prolonged neural blockade and systemic LA toxicity (LAST) may occur.

The safe performance of regional anesthesia requires a thorough knowledge and understanding of LA pharmacology. There are a number of important pharmacologic properties of LAs in pediatric patients, especially neonates and infants (<1 year of age) that differ from the adult patient.

This chapter will highlight these important differences, as well as the basic principles of LA pharmacology.

Mechanism of action (pharmacodynamics)

LAs exist in two forms, ionized hydrophilic (BH^+) and non-ionized lipophilic (B). The non-ionized lipophilic form passes through the hydrophobic cell membrane rapidly. Once in the cytoplasm, the non-ionized and ionized fractions reach equilibrium ($B + H^+ \rightleftharpoons BH^+$). The ionized fraction is active and binds to the membrane-bound, voltage-gated sodium channels involved in the propagation of signaling. The sodium channel exists in one of three conformational states. The channel is closed when "resting" or "inactivated," and open when "activated." The membrane potential affects the conformational state, with depolarization leading to more open channels. LAs have a greater affinity for the sodium channel when it is in the "activated" conformation; thus, when nerve

signals fire more frequently, LA affinity for the sodium channel increases. This results in an increased portion of blocked channels (Figure 3.1).

The channels become activated after chemical, mechanical, or electrical stimuli (i.e. pain impulse). As sodium ions enter into the cell an action potential is generated that is conducted as a nerve impulse (Figure 3.2). LAs bind and inhibit the sodium channels from inside the cell via reversible ionic interactions with the alpha subunit of the sodium channel. It is the ionized fraction that binds with higher affinity and dissociates from the channel subunit at a slower rate. This prevents cell membrane depolarization by blocking sodium ions from entering into the cell and preventing the channel from changing its conformation. The resulting interruption of signal conduction blocks pain transmission and can also lead to motor blockade.

LA action is not limited to peripheral nerve cells. They also affect the myocardium and the central nervous system (CNS). For example, lidocaine has antiarrhythmic properties. At low levels, lidocaine is an anticonvulsant (Mazoit and Dalens, 2004). In toxic doses, however, LAs can lead to adverse CNS events and even cardiovascular collapse.

Sensitivity to blockade

The physical characteristics of peripheral nerve fibers determine sensitivity to blockade by LAs. Sensitivity to LAs is inversely proportional to the increasing diameter, degree of myelination, and conduction velocity. Sensitivity of the nerve to LA blockade is decreased with increasing nerve diameter and increased conduction velocity. Motor nerves are the least sensitive to the effects of LAs as they are large in diameter, have higher conduction velocities, and are myelinated. Sensory fibers are smaller than motor fibers, with some myelinated and some unmyelinated, and thus more sensitive

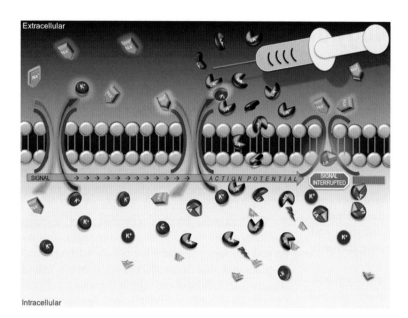

Figure 3.1 Mechanism of action of local anesthetics (LA) at the sodium channel with subsequent blocking of neural transmission. Normal neural transmission is dependent on sodium (Na⁺) influx through Na⁺ channels with potassium (K⁺) outflow restoring resting membrane potential. This pathway is blocked by LA acting at these channels. LA enters the cell in the non-ionized form and is in equilibrium with hydrogen (H⁺) ions with the ionized form active at the sodium channel.

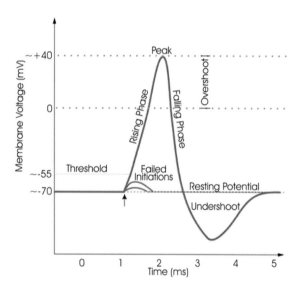

Figure 3.2 Neural action potential. Sodium channels open with subsequent sodium ion influx once the membrane potential voltage reaches −55 mV (threshold). Once the voltage of +40 mV is reached, potassium channels open with the outflow of potassium ions restoring the membrane potential. (Copyright © Synaptitude 2005. Permission is granted to copy, distribute and/or modify this document under the terms of the GNU Free Documentation License, Version 1.3 or any later version published by the Free Software Foundation; with no Invariant Sections, no Front-Cover Texts, and no Back-Cover Texts. A copy of the license is included in the section entitled "GNU Free Documentation License.")

to LAs than motor nerves. Sympathetic, autonomic fibers are small and unmyelinated, rendering them first to be blocked by LAs during neuraxial anesthesia.

Local anesthetic agents

LAs are classified based on their chemical structure. Each LA has an intermediate chain linkage that binds an aromatic group to a tertiary amine. This linkage exists as either an amino-ester or amino-amide bond (Figure 3.3). Ester LAs include chloroprocaine, cocaine, procaine, and tetracaine. Amide LAs include lidocaine, mepivacaine, bupivacaine, ropivacaine, and levobupivacaine.

Amide LAs are longer acting as a result of protein binding and hepatic metabolism, and are typically more suitable for regional techniques.

Potency, onset of action, and duration are pharmacologic principles to consider with LA administration (Table 3.1). Potency refers to the affinity of the LA for the lipid cell membrane of the neuron. More lipid soluble agents have higher potency and higher affinity for binding sodium channels.

Onset of action relates to the pKa of a drug, which is the pH at which the non-ionized form and ionized form are in equal concentration. The ratio of ionized to non-ionized is given by the Henderson–Hasselbalch equation: $pKa = pH + \log[B]/[BH^+]$. The non-ionized form passes through the membrane into the neuron.

Table 3.1 Summary of local anesthetic (LA) potency, onset, and duration of action

Potency	Refers to a LA's affinity for sodium-channel binding Higher lipid solubility = increased potency Affected by nerve diameter and myelination
Onset of action	Related to the pKa of a LA Decreased pKa = increased non-ionized fraction of LA present and more rapid onset Sodium bicarbonate can be added to commercially prepared acidic LA solutions to quicken onset
Duration of action	Increased lipid solubility = increased duration Vasoconstriction = increased duration Epinephrine can be added to increase duration

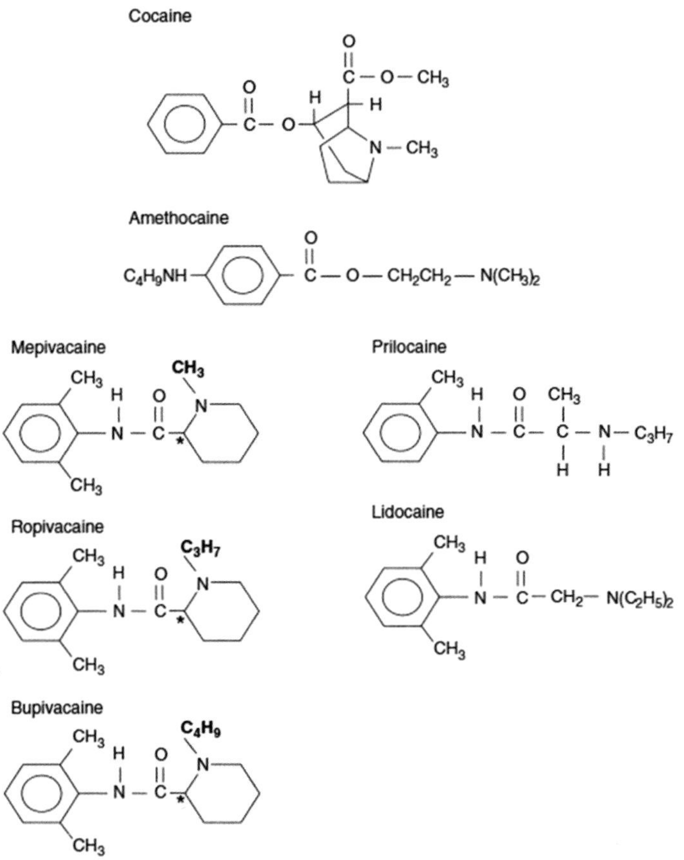

Figure 3.3 Chemical structure of different local anesthetics. Cocaine and amethocaine (tetracaine) are esters. The remainder are amides which have an NH functional group in the intermediate chain linkage. (Reproduced with permission from Peck TE, Hill S. (2008) *Pharmacology for Anaesthesia and Intensive Care*, 3rd edn. Cambridge: Cambridge University Press.)

At a low pKa, less of the ionized fraction and more of the non-ionized fraction is present, allowing for more rapid onset. The concentration and volume also affect the onset. While 3% chloroprocaine has a high pKa, it has a rapid onset secondary to a high concentration (Berde and Strichartz, 2010). The high concentration allows for quick diffusion into the cell. In addition, nerve fiber diameter and myelination affect drug potency.

The duration of action of LAs is also related to lipid solubility. The higher the lipid solubility the longer the duration of action, because of slower systemic absorption from the injection site. More lipophilic LAs have a higher degree of tissue binding, which inhibits systemic absorption. The intrinsic vasoconstrictive properties of ropivacaine also prolong its duration of action.

Additives are sometimes used to speed onset and increase duration of blockade. First, LAs are weak bases, but are prepared as acidic solutions to maintain stability. The addition of sodium bicarbonate at the time of the block shortens the onset by increasing the pH and thus increasing the lipophilic portion of the drug ($B.HCl + HCO_3^- \rightleftharpoons B + H_2CO_3 + Cl^-$). The addition of sodium bicarbonate to a LA may shorten the onset of peripheral and epidural nerve blocks by 3–5 minutes (Stoelting and Hillier, 2006).

Another commonly used additive is epinephrine. Epinephrine can increase duration of blockade of certain LAs secondary to vasoconstriction. The vasoconstriction decreases systemic absorption; it can especially impact neonates and children who have higher cardiac output. Some practitioners caution against using epinephrine with epidural anesthesia in children given the potential to cause spinal cord ischemia (Berde and Greco, 2012).

Protein binding

Amide LAs bind to serum proteins, mainly alpha-1 acid glycoprotein (AAG). The degree of protein binding varies for the different LAs, with lidocaine having 65% protein binding in adults and bupivacaine and ropivacaine having 95% protein binding (Mazoit and Dalens, 2004). Also, the amount of AAG in the serum varies between children less than 1 year old and that in older children or adults. The concentration increases over the first year from 0.2–0.3g/L at birth to 0.7–1.0g/l at 1 year, which is same concentration as in adults (Mazoit and Dalens, 2004). Thus, in children less than 1 year of age, more drug exists in the unbound free form, which increases the potential for systemic toxicity. It is absolutely necessary to understand that infants have decreased LA protein binding secondary to lower AAG levels. The traditional concept is that lower concentrations of AAG result in increased free drug (LA) availability and, hence, increased risk of toxicity (Polaner et al., 2010). However, as there is a dynamic interaction between free LA in equilibrium with the fraction bound to proteins and to the tissues, the clinical significance of lower AAG concentrations is unclear (Lönnqvist, 2012). As part of the acute phase response, AAG concentrations have been shown to increase after stress and surgery in infants, further reducing the effects of protein binding as a factor in LAST. Caution is advised when directly translating the maximum allowable dose of LAs adults to clinical

use in infants. It is recommended that doses should be reduced in very young infants (Dalens, 2010).

In addition to AAG binding, LAs bind to human serum albumin. This interaction holds less clinical significance as LA affinity is much lower for albumin than AAG, especially at normal clinical levels. Albumin can become a clinically significant buffer when AAG sites become saturated at toxic doses (Mazoit and Dalens, 2004). In addition to serum proteins, amide LAs also bind to red blood cells. Twenty to thirty percent of the drug in circulation is bound to erythrocytes. Since erythrocyte-binding sites are not saturated in clinical situations, this binding can also act as a buffer when toxic levels arise (Mazoit and Dalens, 2004). Red blood count binding might be more significant in neonates as they naturally have polycythemia and macrocythemia, allowing for more LA binding to help prevent toxicity (Mazoit and Dalens, 2004).

Pharmacokinetics: absorption, distribution, clearance
Systemic absorption

Absorption of LAs into systemic circulation depends on blood flow; thus, absorption is different for neuraxial blocks and peripheral nerve blocks depending on blood flow to the different injection sites. Absorption from highest to lowest occurs as follows: intravenous > tracheal > intercostal > caudal > paracervical > epidural > brachial plexus > sciatic > subcutaneous. The presence of vasoconstrictors, such as epinephrine, decrease LA absorption by constricting local blood vessels and uptake of LA into the circulation. Limiting circulation to the injection site will increase the duration of the block, especially with shorter-acting drugs such as lidocaine. In addition, ropivacaine has intrinsic vasoconstrictor properties that may decrease absorption. The LAs that are highly protein bound (bupivacaine, ropivacaine, levobupivacaine) have slower absorption rates than less protein-bound agents (lidocaine). Other factors affecting absorption include the dose and volume of the LA.

Cardiac output also plays an important part in systemic absorption. The higher the cardiac output, the higher the systemic absorption. Since children, especially neonates, have higher cardiac output than adults, they also have increased systemic absorption and risk for toxicity.

Distribution

Infants have a higher extracellular fluid content than adults and, thus, a higher volume of distribution. This may play a protective role by lowering peak plasma concentration after a single injection of LA. This likely counteracts the risk of toxicity that results from increased cardiac output and absorption in infants and young children after a single dose. However, with repeated dosing or infusions, accumulation of plasma concentrations can occur (Dalens, 2010).

Clearance: metabolism and elimination

Ester LAs are metabolized rapidly by plasma pseudocholinesterase in both adults and children, including neonates (Berde, 2004). The metabolites are water soluble and undergo renal excretion. The esters, procaine and benzocaine, have a metabolite, para-amino benzoic acid (PABA), which can cause allergic reactions. Cocaine is unique amongst the ester LAs. It undergoes slow hydrolysis (Dalens, 2010), and is partially metabolized in the liver with some unchanged renal elimination. While plasma cholinesterase activity is decreased in neonates and infants, it typically does not cause clinically significant adverse events (Dalens, 2010).

Amide LAs, contrary to esters, are metabolized in the liver by the cytochrome P450 system. These enzymes are immature at birth. Thus, neonates and infants clear amide LAs slower. Because plasma clearance is decreased and elimination half-life is increased in infants, repeated doses could cause increased LA levels (Dalens, 2010).

Local anesthetic systemic toxicity (LAST)

LAST is rare in infants and children. Please refer to Chapter 4 for the management of LAST.

Certain physiologic states increase the risk of LA systemic cardiac toxicity in all patients, including preexisting cardiac pathology, acidosis, hypothermia, electrolyte disorders, and hypoxia (Mazoit and Dalens, 2004). Acidosis increases the fraction of an amide LA in the ionized unbound form, which is the form responsible for systemic toxicity. In addition, prilocaine can cause methemoglobinemia via oxidation of hemoglobin, especially in neonates with circulating fetal hemogloblin (Stoelting and Hillier, 2006).

Certain physiologic characteristics make pediatric patients, especially neonates and infants, more susceptible to toxicity than adults (Table 3.2). When compared to an adult patient, children have an increased volume of distribution, a higher resting heart rate, an increased cardiac output and a less efficient P450 liver enzyme system. Decreased protein binding secondary to lower levels of AAG in infants leads to increased levels of unbound amide LAs. Postoperative increases in AAG in very young infants might not increase enough to counteract the intrinsic low levels (Meunier et al., 2011). Also, increased resting heart rates can increase risk since LAs bind more avidly to the sodium channel when it is active and firing. This phenomenon, known as "rate dependence," explains why infants and children are more prone to the toxicity with bupivacaine or ropivacaine (Mazoit and Dalens, 2004).

Of the LAs, the inadvertent intravenous injection of bupivacaine is one of the most dangerous in adults

Table 3.2 Physiologic characteristics leading to increased risk of LAST in children (especially infants/neonates)

Physiologic characteristic	Clinical implication
Decreased protein binding (lower levels of AAG) in infants	Increased plasma levels of unbound amide LA
Increased resting heart rates	LA bind more avidly to activated sodium channels; may increase risk of cardiac toxicity
Increased cardiac output	Increased systemic absorption→ leads to increased plasma levels of LA
Immature P450 enzymes	Slower metabolism of amide LA Risk of toxicity with repeated injections
Increased extracellular fluid and volume of distribution	Risk of drug accumulation with repeated doses or infusions (while a single dose actually results in a low plasma concentration)

AAG, alpha-1 acid glycoprotein; LA, local anesthetic; LAST, local anesthetic systemic toxicity (LAST).

and children. Bupivacaine binds with high affinity to cardiac sodium channels for a longer duration than other agents. Its binding with other channels in the myocardium, including potassium and calcium channels, may lead to cardiovascular collapse and even death.

Some amide LAs, including bupivacaine, exist as enantiomers, and it is important to note that the (R)–(+) enantiomer of bupivacaine is considered more toxic than the (S)–(–) enantiomer. Ropivacaine and levobupivacaine consist purely of the S-enantiomer. These drugs have less cardiac toxicity and neurotoxicity. They result in more sensory blockade and less motor blockade than bupivacaine. However, the risk of toxicity does exist even with these "safer" forms of the LAs.

In addition to systemic toxicity, the potential also exists for local toxicity at the injection site with neuraxial anesthesia in pediatric patients. Cauda equina syndrome has occurred with tetracaine and lidocaine injection, while transient neurologic symptoms (TNS) have been reported after the use of spinal lidocaine and bupivacaine. In addition, epinephrine use in caudal and lumbar epidural anesthesia at higher concentrations (1:200 000) can theoretically lead to neurologic complications caused by decreased spinal cord perfusion (Mazoit and Dalens, 2004).

Summary

The use of ultrasound to guide regional anesthesia in children is becoming more widely utilized. Ultrasound use likely helps to decrease the risk of adverse events, including inadvertent intravascular injection and, thus, systemic toxicity. It does not, however, remove the risk entirely. Ultrasound-guided blocks also require smaller volumes of LA for successful blockade. Practitioners must be aware of the unique LA pharmacology in children as well as the signs and symptoms of toxicity. Protocols should be in place for the treatment of toxicity at all sites where regional anesthesia is performed. Compared to adults, important pharmacological considerations exist in children, which increase their risk of systemic toxicity. These differences must be considered when performing regional anesthesia in children. In summary, these differences include:

- Delayed nerve fiber myelination resulting in quicker onset of neural blockade – less concentrated LA may reduce toxicity risk (Berde and Strichartz, 2010).
- Less protein binding of amide LA secondary to lower levels of AAG increases the unbound form of the drug and may increase LAST risk.
- Increased cardiac output leads to increased absorption from the injection site.
- Faster resting heart rates, which can increase toxicity risk since LA binds more avidly to sodium channels in the activated state.
- Increased extracellular fluids (and, thus, volume of distribution) resulting in decreased plasma concentrations after a single dose of LA but with drug accumulation after repeated doses or infusions.
- Immature P450 system results in decreased metabolism and clearance of amide LA, and repeated injections can, therefore, cause toxicity.
- Children may have cardiac toxicity before or without CNS symptoms of LAST.
- Neonates have fetal hemoglobin in the circulation increasing the risk of methemoglobinemia with prilocaine usage.

Suggested reading

Berde C. (2004) Local anesthetics in infants and children: an update. *Paediatr Anaesth.* 14,387–93.

Berde C, Greco C. (2012) Pediatric regional anesthesia: drawing inferences on safety from prospective registries and case reports. *Anesth Analg.* 115 (6), 1259–62.

Berde C, Strichartz G. (2010) Local anesthetics. In Miller, R. ed. *Miller's Anesthesia*, 7th edn. Philadelphia, PA: Churchill Livingstone.

Dalens B. (2010) Regional anesthesia in children. In Miller, R. ed. *Miller's Anesthesia*, 7th edn. Philadelphia, PA: Churchill Livingstone.

Davis P, Bosenberg A, Davidson A, et al. (2011) Pharmacology of pediatric anesthesia. In Davis P, Cladis F, Motoyama E. eds. *Smith's Anesthesia for Infants and Children*, 8th edn. Philadelphia, PA: Elsevier Mosby.

Lönnqvist PA. (2012) Toxicity of local anesthetic drugs: a pediatric perspective. *Paediatr Anaesth.* 22,39–43.

Marhofer P, Frickey N. (2006) Ultrasonographic guidance in pediatric regional anesthesia part 1: theoretical. *Paediatr Anaesth.* 16,1008–18.

Mazoit JX, Dalens B. (2004) Pharmacokinetics of local anaesthetics in infants and children. *Clin Pharmacokinet.* 43(1),17–32.

Meunier JX, Goujard E, Dubousset AM, Kamran S. (2011) Pharmacokinetics of bupivacaine after continuous epidural infusion in infants with and without biliary atresia. *Anesthesiology.* 95(1),87–95.

Neal J, Bernards C, Butterworth J, et al. (2010) ASRA practice advisory on local anesthetic systemic toxicity. *Reg Anesth Pain Med.* 35(2),152–61.

Polaner DM, Zuk J, Luong K, Pan Z. (2010). Positive intravascular test dose criteria in children during total intravenous anesthesia with propofol and remifentanil are different than during inhaled anesthesia. *Anesth Analg.* 110,41–5.

Polaner DM, Taenzer A, Walker B, et al. (2012) Pediatric regional and network (PRAN) a multi-institutional study of the use and incidence of complications in pediatric regional anesthesia. *Anesth Analg.* 115(6),1352–64.

Presley J, Chyka P. (2013) Intravenous lipid emulsion to reverse acute drug toxicity in pediatric patients. *Ann Pharmacother.* 47,735–43.

Roberts S. (2006) Ultrasonographic guidance in pediatric regional anesthesia. Part 2: techniques. *Paediatr Anaesth.* 16,1112–24.

Stoelting R, Hillier S. (2006) *Pharmacology & Physiology in Anesthetic Practice*, 4th edn. Philadelphia, PA: Lippincott Williams & Wilkins.

Management of complications of regional anesthesia

Immanuel Hennessy and Stephen Mannion

Introduction

Regional anesthesia in children is safe. Serious complications such as nerve injury, systemic toxicity, serious infections, and visceral or dural punctures are very rare.

Complications following regional anesthesia can be minimized through good clinical practice, and there is increasing evidence that ultrasonography may play an increasing role in further enhancing safety (Griffin and Nicholls, 2010).

Recently three large databases have provided prospective data on the complications of regional anesthesia in children. The Pediatric Regional Anesthesia Network (PRAN) study (Polaner et al., 2012), the French-Language Society of Pediatric Anesthesiologists (ADARPEF) survey (Ecoffey et al., 2010), and the National Paediatric Epidural Audit (NPEA) from the UK and Ireland (Llewellyn and Moriarty, 2007), together have reported on the complication rates relating to 56 682 regional anesthetic procedures in children.

Overall the reported risk of serious complications in these studies has been shown to be very low. Notably there were no deaths from regional anesthesia reported in any of these studies. There was only 1 case of morbidity with effects lasting greater than 1 year. This case was reported in the NPEA and involved a 4-month-old child, who had a partial neurologic deficit still present 1 year after an epidural drug error. The incidence of serious complications in the French and American databases ranged from 0.12 to 0.15%. In all these cases, resolution of the complication occurred by the studies' follow-up times of 3 months (PRAN) or 1 year (ADARPEF).

These data are reassuring as regards the safety profile of regional anesthesia in children; however, they should not lead to complacency as the risk is never zero (Boretsky, 2014).

This chapter will discuss the types of major complications after regional anesthesia in children and describe the management of each of these.

Local anesthetic systemic toxicity

In children, local anesthetic systemic toxicity (LAST) following regional anesthesia is an extremely rare but potentially life-threatening condition. The risk of developing LAST is estimated to be 0 to 2:10 000 from prospective databases (PRAN/ADARPEF/NPEA). This is similar to the risk of LAST in adults, which was recently estimated to be 0.37:10 000 (Ecoffey et al., 2014).

LAST occurs when excessive local anesthetic (LA) is present in blood resulting in LA concentrations that cause cardiac and central nervous system (CNS) toxicity. General anesthesia can mask the early clinical signs of LAST in children, although the incidence is four times less than in awake or sedated children (Taenzer et al., 2014a). Younger children may present with non-specific symptoms, such as restlessness, agitation, and irritability, whereas older awake children may give a more classical description of CNS toxicity (perioral numbness, metallic taste, tinnitus, restlessness, headache). Contrary to traditional teaching cardiovascular system (CVS) effects can occur before or in the absence of any CNS symptoms.

Mechanism of action

The mechanism of action of CNS toxicity is through inhibition of inhibitory CNS neural pathways by blocking sodium channels. This is followed by inhibition of excitatory pathways at high drug concentrations resulting in generalized CNS depression. CVS effects are as a result of the action of LA on cardiac fast sodium channels, slowing cardiac depolarization by blocking the inactivated channel. This increase in

Ultrasound-Guided Regional Anesthesia in Children, ed. Mannion et al. Published by Cambridge University Press.
© Cambridge University Press 2015.

conduction times is manifested as prolonged P–R intervals and QRS duration. LA also acts at L-type calcium channels, resulting in both slower conduction and depressed myocardial contractility (Dippenaar, 2007). Different LA drugs have a different C_{max} (maximum concentration) in blood after which toxic effects are more likely to occur. C_{max} varies depending on whether blood sampling is venous or arterial. LA concentrations may rise in blood depending on a number of factors.

The most rapid rise to C_{max} is from direct intravascular injection with a more rapid onset of toxicity with intra-arterial compared to intravenous injection.

Prevention

LAST is a potential life-threatening emergency. The risk of systemic toxicity can be minimized by careful attention to the maximum permitted doses of LA, the addition of epinephrine, slow and fractionated injection, regular aspiration before each injection, the avoidance of injection if blood is detected, and the use of smaller volumes of LA. Electocardiographic (ECG) monitoring is mandatory. The use of ultrasound for regional anesthesia in children permits the use of smaller volumes of LA in a number of blocks (Boretsky, 2014).

Ultrasound also allows visualization of vascular structures. A recent meta-analysis found a sixfold reduction in vascular puncture comparing ultrasound-guided with nerve stimulator block techniques in adults (Abrahams et al., 2009). There were no cases of systemic LA toxicity or neural injury in either group. However, the available data in children does not demonstrate similar findings and there were no cases of vascular puncture or neural injury reported in 5 studies, which randomized a total of 276 children to either ultrasound or nerve stimulator-guided blocks (Marhofer et al., 2004; Oberndorfer et al., 2007; De José María et al., 2008; Ponde and Diwan, 2009; Ponde et al., 2013). Any safety advantages of ultrasound over nerve stimulator techniques on vascular or neural outcomes have not as yet been adequately demonstrated in children (Rubin et al., 2009). Nevertheless, any technique that reduces the factors known to be associated with LAST is welcome.

Recognition of intravascular injection in pediatrics is difficult for a number of reasons. The early clinical symptoms such as confusion, drowsiness, perioral paresthesia, and tinnitus will be absent because of concurrent general anesthesia. Aspiration of smaller diameter needles and catheters make recognition of an intravascular placement difficult in children. A series of 742 caudal and epidural blocks found an intravenous injection rate of 5.6% with a positive aspiration of blood of only 0.8%. (Fisher et al., 1997).

Recent studies have shown a 0.05% incidence of transient cardiac toxicity (Ecoffey et al., 2010) and, overall, vascular punctures or positive test doses appear to be more common in single shot central blocks and catheter blocks compared with single shot peripheral blocks (Table 4.1).

A test dose of LA with epinephrine 0.5 µg/kg is one method to detect a positive intravenous injection. A positive test dose is an increase in heart rate by greater than 10 beats per minute above baseline occurring within 1 minute of injection (Ecoffey 2012). Heart rate changes alone in an anesthetized child may miss up to 36% of intravenous injections. An increase in T-wave amplitude can detect up to 94% of positive intravenous injections (Varghese et al., 2009). These parameters are unreliable if total intravenous anesthesia (TIVA) and remifentanil anesthesia is used; in these cases an increase in blood pressure should be monitored for (Polaner et al., 2010).

Different LAs have different pharmacokinetics and also differing levels of toxicity. Racemic bupivacaine is the most cardiac toxic followed by its S-enantiomer, levobupivacaine, and then ropivacaine (Lönnqvist, 2012). Short-acting lidocaine usually presents with CNS toxicity (Figure 4.1). The systemic absorption will also depend on the site of injection, with the addition of epinephrine (1:100 000–200 000) reducing the peak plasma concentrations (Chalkiadis et al., 2013). The speed of the injection and the total dose will be the major determinants of whether systemic toxicity occurs or not.

A safe C_{max} of LA can be achieved with adherence to dosing guidelines for neonates, infants, and children (Berde, 1993). Dosing for ropivacaine and levobupivacaine generally follow those established for bupivacaine (Table 4.2), although they are less toxic. In infants, ropivacaine undergoes slower absorption that may result in increased peak plasma concentration. For continuous infusions, however, ropivacaine is recommended as having the safest therapeutic index (Dalens, 2006).

Care should be taken in children with hepatic, renal, or cardiac conditions that may effect LA doses through altered pharmacokinetics, and reduced metabolism and elimination. In particular, infants aged less than 1 year, and especially those less than 6 months, carry a higher risk of developing systemic toxicity. This is as a result of factors including an immature liver, lower levels of pseudocholinesterase,

21

Table 4.1 Summary of cardiovascular, neurologic, and infectious adverse effects in 14 917 blocks from the PRAN study

Block type	No. of blocks	Positive test dose	Vascular puncture	CVS event	Neuro event	Infectious event
Neuraxial single shot	6210	18	38	2*	0	0
Neuraxial catheter	2946	13	33	1	3[†]	32[‡]
Lower limb single shot	2307	NR	NR	NR	0	0
Lower limb catheter	544	0	10	0	1[§]	3[¶]
Upper limb single shot	455	0	0	0	0	0
Upper limb catheter	26	0	0	0	0	0
Head and neck single shot	556	0	0	0	0	0
Truncal single shot	1112	1	0	0	0	0
Truncal catheter	24	0	0	0	0	0
Ilioinguinal single shot	737	0	1	0	0	0

* One case was of hypotension post-spinal anesthesia in a teenager.
[†] All cases involved lumbar/thoracic epidural catheters, and all neurologic events were transient and recovered in the immediate post-operative period.
[‡] Only 3/32 cases required antibiotics with no long-term sequelae.
[§] Transient neurologic symptoms after lumbar plexus block, which resolved within 3 months and may have been present preoperatively.
[¶] Three cases of superficial infections (one each for femoral, sciatic, and popliteal).
NR: not reported in the original study – 33 adverse events of which 14 were block failure. The remaining 19 cases were not described, but no complications were reported that resulted in patient harm or sequelae.
Truncal includes paravertebral, intercostal, and abdominal blocks
There were no cases of LAST or of neurologic injury lasting more than 3 months.
CVS, cardiovascular system; LAST, local anesthetic systemic toxicity; PRAN, Pediatric Regional Anesthesia Network.

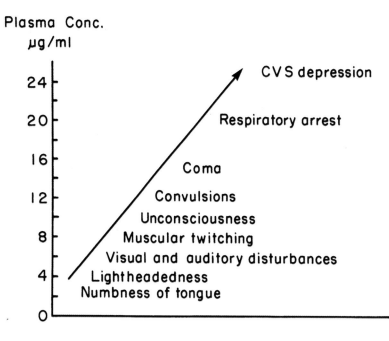

Figure 4.1 Schematic of toxic clinical symptoms with increasing plasma lidocaine concentrations. This classical hierachy of symptoms presents in less than 50% of cases of lidocaine toxicity. (Reproduced with permission of the author from Cousins MJ, et al. *Cousins and Bridenbaugh's Neural Blockade in Clinical Anesthesia and Pain Medicine*, 4th edn. Philadelphia, PA: Wolter Kluwers and Lippincott Williams & Wilkins, p. 115.)

Table 4.2 Recommended doses of local anesthetics in children

Drug	Bolus	Infusion <3 months of age[*]	Infusion <1 year and >3 months of age[*]	Infusion >1 year of age[*]
Bupivacaine	2 mg/kg[†]	0.2 mg/kg/h	0.3 mg/kg/h	0.4 mg/kg/h
Levobupivacaine	2 mg/kg	0.2 mg/kg/h	0.3 mg/kg/h	0.4 mg/kg/h
Ropivacaine	2 mg/kg	0.2 mg/kg/h	0.3 mg/kg/h	0.4 mg/kg/h
Mepivacaine	4 mg/kg	NA	NA	NA
Lidocaine plain	4 mg/kg	NA	NA	NA
Lidocaine + epinephrine	7 mg/kg	NA	NA	NA

Dosages should be based on lean body mass (LBM). An equation for lean body mass based on extracellular volume (ECV) is: eLBM = 3.5 × ECV + 2.0; where ECV = $weight^{0.6469}$ × $height^{0.7236}$ × 0.02154. Weight in kilograms, height in centimeters (Peters et al., 2011). In practical terms, LBM is approximately 60% of total body weight (TBW).
NA, not applicable.
[*] Infusions for >48 h result in increased plasma concentrations especially in neonates.
[†] For children <5 kg, a bolus dose of 1.25 mg/kg bupivacaine has been recommended.

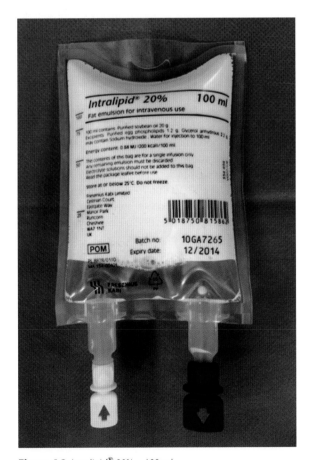

Figure 4.2 Intralipid® 20% – 100 ml.

and reduced protein binding of LA, because of low plasma concentrations of alpha-1 acid glycoprotein (AAG) (Lönnqvist, 2012).

Management

Any suspicion of LAST requires early detection and stopping the administration of the drug. Senior help should be called for and supportive care initiated. A recommended management plan is presented in Box 4.1.

The greatest change in the management of LAST has been the use of intravenous lipid emulsions, in most cases 20% Intralipid® (Weinberg et al., 1998) (Figure 4.2). Lipid emulsions have been particularly effective in reversing the CVS effects of bupivacaine toxicity, but have been successfully used clinically to treat CVS toxicity secondary to most LAs (Weinberg, 2012). The knowledge of how lipid emulsions work is incomplete. Mechanisms proposed include the concept of a "lipid sink," an alternative energy substrate or metabolic effect, or a combination of both (Kuo and Akpa, 2012).

Regardless of the mechanism of action, lipid emulsion has been successfully used to treat LAST with CVS effects in children (Presley and Chyka, 2013). In children, lipid emulsion was effective for treating LAST secondary to regional anesthesia-related bupivacaine, ropivacaine, and lidocaine

Suggested use of Intralipid® in the management of local anesthetic systemic toxicity (LAST) in children

A. Establish secure airway and give 100% oxygen (patient may require respiratory ventilatory support and tracheal intubation)
B. Manage cardiac arrest by following standard pediatric advanced life support guidelines (PALS), including use of epinephrine
C. Treat seizures with barbiturates, benzodiazepines, or propofol
D. Administer a 2 ml/kg initial bolus of Intralipid® 20%
E. Repeat initial bolus twice every 3 minutes if cardiovascular stability not resored
F. Commence infusion of 0.25 ml/kg/h Intralipid® 20%
G. Increase infusion to 0.5 ml/kg/h if cardiovascular stability not restored or deterioration
H. Total maximum dose is 10 ml/kg. This allows a total infusion time of 16 minutes if maintained at 0.25 ml/kg/h

systemic absorption, as well as a case of accidental orally ingested dibucaine.

Safe dosing limits for lipid resuscitation are important to establish in neonates and children because complications (fat embolism, triglyceridemia, pancreatitis, ventilation–perfusion mismatch) from lipid overload have been reported in neonates and young children (Barson et al., 1978; Presley and Chyka, 2013; Shenoy et al., 2014). In adults both the Association of Anaesthetists of Great Britain and Ireland (AAGBI) and the American Society of Regional Anesthesia (ASRA) have published guidelines on the use of Intralipid® for LAST in adults. Currently there are no official guidelines for children. Both the AAGBI and ASRA recommend an initially bolus of 1.5 ml/kg of 20% Intralipid®. Bolus doses of 2 ml/kg and 3 ml/kg have been used successfully in a neonate and a 12-year-old child respectively (Ludot et al., 2008; Shah S. et al., 2009). However, doses up to 5 ml/kg have been recommended, with repeated boluses up to 10 ml/kg in the absence of cardiac output (Gregory and Andropoulos, 2012; Shah RD and Suresh, 2013). The AAGBI and ASRA guidelines vary in terms of the number of repeat boluses (2 vs. 1) and the maximum permissible amount (12 ml/kg vs. 10 ml/kg). Both recommend the commencement of an

infusion of 0.25 ml/kg/h, which can be increased to 0.5 ml/kg/h if there's no effect or clinical deterioration. In children there have been no reports to date of the use of a continuous infusion. It is important that the other components of resuscitation for children, including the early administration of epinephrine, are followed (de Queiroz Siqueira et al., 2014).

Infection

Infection after regional anesthesia in children is rare, particularly if single shot peripheral nerve blockade (PNB) is performed. Nevertheless strict aseptic precautions should always be taken. Guidelines have been produced by the ASRA and other national organizations, including SFAR (Société Française d'Anesthésie et de Réanimation) in France.

Infection after catheter-based techniques is rare, but bacterial colonization of indwelling epidural and caudal catheters has a reported incidence of 6–35% (Ecoffey, 2012).The presence and duration of an indwelling catheter increases the risk of infection – particularly if left in place for longer than 5 days (Strafford et al., 1995; Llewellyn and Moriarty, 2007).

Infection associated with regional anesthesia has been classified as superficial or deep, with deep infections having potentially serious implications. The PRAN database showed no deep neuraxial infections in 9156 neuraxial blocks. The incidence of serious infection was 0 to 13:10 000 (95% confidence interval (CI)) in this study, with other studies having similar findings (Strafford et al., 1995; Llewellyn and Moriarty, 2007; Polaner et al., 2012).

There were 28 complications related to infection in 10 633 epidural catheters in the NPEA study (Llewellyn and Moriarty, 2007). Superficial infection accounted for 25 of the 28, with the majority being caused by gram-positive organisms, giving a superficial infection incidence of 0.3%. Of the 3 deep infections, there were 2 cases of epidural abscess and 1 child presented with meningeal signs, giving a deep infection incidence of 0.02%. Another long-term study of epidural catheters gave a lower overall incidence of infection at 0.06%; however, this study had strict inclusion criteria which did not count induration/erythema at the catheter exit site that spontaneously resolved. A study of peripheral nerve catheters found 1 uncomplicated case of cellulitis that responded to antibiotics out of 226 children (Ganesh et al., 2007). The rate of catheter-related infections is lower in children than in adults (Dadure and Capdevila, 2012).

Management

Primary prevention of infection is important. Skin preparation and adherence to strict aseptic precautions may reduce the risk of infection (Strafford et al., 1995). Alcohol may be useful for transiently decontaminating the skin; however, for bacteria in the deeper skin layers it is recommended by current national society guidelines (ASRA, ASA, AAGBI) that chlorhexidine gluconate (0.5–2.0%) with 70% alcohol solutions is used. Particular care should be taken to ensure that ultrasound probes are sterile prior to use and that a sterile gel is used (Figure 4.3).

Daily monitoring of the catheter insertion site should take place while the catheter is place and for up to 72 hours once it has been removed. This is recommended practice as a number of the reported infections in the NPEA study (including 1 of epidural abscess) presented more than 24 hours after removal of the catheter (Llewellyn and Moriarty, 2007).

Catheter-related infection should be suspected if there are signs of local soft tissue infection/inflammation or systemic infection (raised temperature, raised white cell count or increased C-reactive

protein). If a superficial infection is suspected the catheter should be removed and the tip sent for culture and antibiotic sensitivities. Any local pus should also be cultured and sensitivities determined. Local skin care and antibiotics may be required.

Deep infections may present with fever and signs of systemic infection. Blood cultures should be taken if systemic infection is being considered and intravenous antibiotics started without delay. A surgical opinion should be sought were there is a deep or non-resolving abscess or collection.

The majority of catheter-related infections are caused by *Staphylococcus aureus,* and appropriate antimicrobial agents should be administered with consideration given to using antibiotics active against methicillin-resistant *S. aureus* (MRSA). Gram-negative colonization of caudal catheters in children does occur and, although uncommon, treating a suspected epidural infection from a caudal catheter should include antimicrobials that are effective against gram-negative micro-organisms.

Nerve injury

Nerve injury following regional anesthesia in both pediatric and adult populations is rare. Ultrasound guidance, by demonstrating the needle, nerve, and other structures as well as monitoring the distribution and spread of LA, may improve the safety of regional anesthesia. The visualized needle can also be repositioned with confidence in the case of a malpositioned needle. Despite this theoretical advantage, as yet there is no large prospective randomized controlled trial to support the assertion that ultrasound guidance has a better safety profile over landmark anatomic or nerve stimulating techniques in children (Ecoffey et al. 2014).

Diagnosing paresthesia in infants and non-verbal children is difficult as they may not complain of symptoms. It should be noted that in 14 917 techniques captured in the PRAN database, there were no permanent nerve injuries. There was 1 case of dysesthesia following a lumbar plexus block reported that resolved within 3 months, and 3 cases of transient post-operative paresthesias after neuraxial catheters (Table 4.1). The incidence of nerve injury following neuraxial anesthesia in children has been reported as 6:10 000 (Llewellyn and Moriarty, 2007). This figure is similar to other studies (Dahlgren and Torenbrandt, 1995). A retrospective study (Flandin-Blety

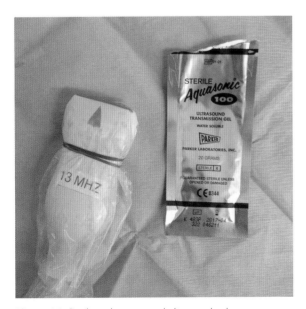

Figure 4.3 Sterile probe cover and ultrasound gel.

and Barrier, 1995) of epidural complications in children reported five severe permanent neurologic events mostly occurring with a loss of resistance to air. Other studies have not shown the same when saline is used (Flandin-Blety and Barrier, 1995; Llewellyn and Moriarty, 2007).

An incidence of peripheral nerve injury in pediatric patients following PNB is not accurately known, but a figure of 2:1000 has been reported in adults (Borgeat and Blumenthal, 2004). Certain blocks in adults have been associated with increased incidence of nerve injury compared to others: interscalene more than axillary brachial plexus block and femoral more than psoas compartment (posterior lumbar plexus) block. However, data from large prospective databases in children do not support these traditional views (Taenzer et al., 2014b).

Management

The modern practice of regional anesthesia aims to avoid nerve injury occurring. Nerve localization techniques, such as ultrasound guidance and nerve stimulation, result in less paresthesia with needle placement and, for some blocks (e.g. interscalene), less nerve injury. This is important in pediatrics as regional blocks usually occur with the patient anesthetized or heavily sedated and, therefore, they cannot communicate whether paresthesia has occurred or if there is pain on injection. Preoperative documentation of any existing neurologic deficits is recommended (e.g. multiple sclerosis, diabetes mellitus, and traumatic injury).

The pressure at which LA is injected is important as pressures in excess of 20–25 lbs/inch^2 (psi) have been shown to cause significant nerve damage in animal studies (dogs) if the needle is within the nerve fascicle. Simple pressure gauges, which connect onto the injecting line, are now available, while it is advisable to avoid syringes less than 10 ml because of the increased pressure on injection because of the smaller area of the syringe plunger relative to the force applied (Pressure = Force/Area). Reducing the dose of LA (volume or concentration) and avoiding vasoconstrictors may also be protective.

Patients should be followed up after any regional technique and a record made of the return of normal sensory and motor function. In the event of a

Table 4.3 Reported complications of regional anesthesia in children

- Failed block
- Local anesthetic systemic toxicity (LAST)
- Infection
- Nerve injury
- Drug error
- Dural puncture
- Colonic puncture
- Bilateral blockade
- Methemoglobinemia secondary to prilocaine
- Hemodynamic effects
- Respiratory compromise (neuraxial opioid infusions)
- Cardiac arrest

neurologic event post the procedure, healthcare staff caring for the child need to be made aware of the need to contact the anesthesiologist if these symptoms/signs become apparent.

Once a nerve injury is reported, the child should be seen urgently and the full extent of the neurologic deficit mapped out. A specialist neurologic opinion may need to be sought to assist with this. It is recommended in cases of documented deficits to discuss the management with a neurologist and/or neurosurgeon/plastic surgeon. Both the anesthesia technique and the surgical procedure may cause or contribute to a post-operative nerve injury and early communication with the surgical team is essential to avoid a blame-game clouding patient management.

In cases of mild or resolving sensory symptoms, informing the patient of the findings and giving reassurance that the prognosis is excellent (99.9% recovery) is sufficient. Ongoing sensory or any motor deficits noted on examination require early neurologic consultation and may warrant magnetic resonance imaging (MRI) or neurophysiologic testing (electromyography (EMG) and nerve conduction studies) to determine the location and extent of nerve injury. Although it takes 14–21 days for neurophysiologic changes to occur after an insult, early testing may be helpful to establish baseline function and rule out any preexisting neurologic condition. Patients with a neurologic deficit should be followed up for 3–6 months, and if there are improvements, conservative treatment is recommended to be continued, which includes physiotherapy. A neurosurgical/plastic surgery opinion should be sought for lesions that have not recovered within the 3–6 month time period as surgical repair may be required in certain cases, but parents of affected children can be reassured that 90% of cases resolve by 1 year.

Conclusion

Complications after regional anesthesia in children are rare – with only a few cases reported in the literature (Table 4.3). However, the use of regional anesthesia in the pediatric population is increasing. Therefore, particular care is needed to ensure this safe profile is maintained and improved upon. We recommend that peripheral nerve catheters should be used in preference to neuraxial catheters whenever possible. Ultrasonography offers many advantages over traditional techniques, including visualization of the nerve and vital structures as well as allowing lower LA volumes for successful blockade. These benefits have not been shown in studies to date to reduce complications in children compared to traditional techniques. Larger trials and prospective databases are needed to determine if the incidence of these rare complications can be further reduced by the use of ultrasonography.

Suggested reading

Abrahams MS, Aziz MF, Fu RF, Horn JL. (2009) Ultrasound guidance compared with electrical neurostimulation for peripheral nerve block: a systematic review and meta-analysis of randomized controlled trials. *Br J Anaesth.* 102,408–17.

Barson AJ, Chistwick ML, Doig CM. (1978) Fat embolism in infancy after intravenous fat infusions. *Arch Dis Child.* 53,218–23.

Berde CB. (1993) Toxicity of local anesthetics in infants and children. *J Pediatr.* 122,S14–20.

Bernards CM, Hadzic A, Suresh S, Neal JM. (2008) Regional anesthesia in anesthetized or heavily sedated patients. *Reg Anesth Pain Med.* 33,449–60.

Boretsky KR. (2014) Regional anesthesia in pediatrics: marching forward. *Curr Opin Anaesthesiol.* 27,556–60.

Borgeat A, Blumenthal S. (2004) Nerve injury and regional anaesthesia. *Curr Opin Anaesthesiol* 17, 417–21.

Chalkiadis GA, Abdullah F, Bjorksten AR, et al. (2013) Absorption characteristics of epidural levobupivacaine with adrenaline and clonidine in children. *Paediatr Anaesth.* 23, 58–67.

Dadure C, Capdevila X. (2012) Peripheral catheter techniques. *Paediatr Anaesth.* 22, 93–101.

Dahlgren N, Torenbrandt K. Neurological complications after anesthesia. A follow-up of 18 000 spinal and epidural anesthetics performed over 3 years. (1995) *Acta Anaesthiol Scand.* 39, 872–88.

Dalens B. (2006) Some current controversies in paediatric regional anaesthesia. *Curr Opin Anaesthesiol.* 19, 301–8.

De José María B, Banús E, Navarro Egea M, et al. (2008) Ultrasound-guided supraclavicular vs. infraclavicular brachial plexus blocks in children. *Paediatr Anaesth.* 18, 838–44.

de Queiroz Siqueira M, Chassard D, Musard H, et al. (2014) Resuscitation with lipid, epinephrine, or both in levobupivacaine-induced cardiac toxicity in newborn piglets. *Br J Anaesth.* 112, 729–34.

Dippenaar JM. (2007) Local anaesthetic toxicity. *SAJAA.*13, 23–28.

Ecoffey C. (2012) Safety in pediatric regional anaesthesia. *Pediatr Anaesth.* 22,25–30.

Ecoffey C, Lacroix F, Giaufré E, Orliaguet G, Courrèges P; Association des Anesthésistes Réanimateurs Pédiatriques d'Expression Française (ADARPEF). (2010) Epidemiology and morbidity of regional anesthesia in children: a follow-up one-year prospective survey of the French-Language Society of Paediatric Anaesthesiologists (ADARPEF). *Paediatr Anaesth.* 20,1061–9.

Ecoffey C, Oger E, Marchand-Maillet F, et al. (2014) Complications associated with 27 031 ultrasound-guided axillary brachial plexus blocks: a web-based survey of 36 French centres. *Eur J Anaesthesiol.* 31,606–10.

Fisher QA, Shaffner DH, Yaster M. (1997) Detection of intravascular injection of regional anaesthetics in children. *Can J Anaesth.* 44,592–8.

Flandin-Blety C, Barrier G. (1995) Accidents following epidural anaesthesia in children.The results of a retrospective study. *Paediatr Anaesth.* 5:41–6.

Ganesh A, Rose JB, Wells L, et al. (2007) Continuous peripheral nerve blockade for inpatient and outpatient postoperative analgesia in children. *Anesth Analg.* 105,1234–42.

27

Gregory GA, Andropoulos DB. (2012) *Pediatric Anesthesia.*, 5th edn. Hoboken, NJ: Wiley Blackwell.

Griffin J, Nicholls B. (2010) Ultrasound in regional anaesthesia. *Anaesthesia.* 65(S1),1–12.

Krane EJ, Dalens BJ, Murat I, Murrell D. (1998) The safety of epidurals placed during general anesthesia. *Reg Anesth Pain Med.* 23,433–8.

Kuo I, Akpa BS. (2013) Validity of the lipid sink as a mechanism for the reversal of local anesthetic systemic toxicity: a physiologically based pharmacokinetic model study. *Anesthesiology.* 118, 1350–61

Lei SY, Hache M, Loepke AW. (2014) Clinical research into anesthetic neurotoxicity: does anesthesia cause neurological abnormalities in humans? *J Neurosurg Anesthesiol.* 26,349–57.

Llewellyn N, Moriarty A. (2007) The national pediatric epidural audit. *Paediatr Anaesth.* 17, 520–33.

Lönnqvist PA. (2012) Toxicity of local anesthetic drugs: a pediatric perspective. *Paediatr Anaesth.* 22,39–43.

Ludot H, Tharin JY, Belouadah M, Mazoit JX, Malinovsky JM. (2008) Successful resuscitation after ropivacaine and lidocaine-induced ventricular arrhythmia following posterior lumbar plexus block in a child. *Anesth Analg.* 106,1572–4.

Luz G, Wieser C, Innerhofer P, et al. (1998) Free and total bupivacaine plasma concentrations after continuous epidural anaesthesia in infants and children. *Paediatr Anaesth.* 8,473–8.

Marhofer P, Sitzwohl C, Greher M, Kapral S. (2004)Ultrasound guidance for infraclavicular brachial plexus anaesthesia in children. *Anaesthesia.* 59,642–6.

Neal JM, Bernards CM, Hadzic A, et al. (2008) ASRA practice advisory on neurologic complications in regional anesthesia and pain medicine. *Reg Anesth Pain Med.* 33,404–15.

Oberndorfer U, Marhofer P, Bösenberg A, et al. (2007) Ultrasonographic guidance for sciatic and femoral nerve blocks in children. *Br J Anaesth.* 98, 797–801.

Peters AM, Snelling HL, Glass DM, Bird NJ. (2011) Estimation of lean body mass in children. *Br J Anaesth.* 106,719–23.

Polaner DM, Zuk J, Luong K, Pan Z. (2010) Positive intravascular test dose criteria in children during total intravenous anesthesia with propofol and remifentanil are different than during inhaled anesthesia. *Anesth Analg.* 110, 41–5.

Polaner DM, Taenzer AH, Walker BJ, et al. (2012) Pediatric Regional Anesthesia Network (PRAN): a multi-institutional study of the use and incidence of complications of pediatric regional anesthesia. *Anesth Analg.* 115,1353–64.

Ponde VC, Diwan S. (2009) Does ultrasound guidance improve the success rate of infraclavicular brachial plexus block when compared with nerve stimulation in children with radial club hands? *Anesth Analg.* 108, 1967–70.

Ponde VC, Desai AP, Shah D. (2013) Comparison of success rate of ultrasound-guided sciatic and femoral nerve block and neurostimulation in children with arthrogryposis multiplex congenita: a randomized clinical trial. *Paediatr Anaesth.* 23,74–8.

Presley JD, Chyka PA. (2013) Intravenous lipid emulsion to reverse acute drug toxicity in pediatric patients. *Ann Pharmacother.* 47,735–43.

Puncuh F, Lampugnani E, Kokki H. (2004) Use of spinal anaesthesia in paediatric patients: a single centre experience with 1132 cases. *Paediatr Anaesth.* 14,564–7.

Rubin K, Sullivan D, Sadhasivam S. (2009) Are peripheral and neuraxial blocks with ultrasound guidance more effective and safe in children? *Paediatr Anaesth.* 19,92–6.

Sethna N, Clendenin D, Athiraaman U, et al. (2010) Incidence of epidural catheter-associated infections and continuous epidural analgesia in children. *Anesthesiology.* 113,224–32

Shah RD, Suresh S. (2013) Applications of regional anaesthesia in paediatrics. *Br J Anaesth.* 111(Suppl. 1),114–24.

Shah S, Gopalakrishnan S, Apuya J, Shah S, Martin T. (2009) Use of Intralipid in an infant with impending cardiovascular collapse due to local anesthetic toxicity. *J Anesth.* 23,439–41.

Shenoy U, Paul J, Antony D. (2014) Lipid resuscitation in pediatric patients – need for caution? *Paediatr Anaesth.* 24,332–4.

Strafford MA, Wilder RT, Berde CB. (1995) The risk of infection from epidural analgesia in children: a review of 1620 cases. *Anesth Analg.* 80,234–8.

Taenzer AH, Walker BJ, Bosenberg AT, et al. (2014a) Asleep versus awake: does it matter? Pediatric regional block complications by patient state: a report from the Pediatric Regional Anesthesia Network. *Reg Anesth Pain Med.* 39,279–83.

Taenzer AH, Walker BJ, Bosenberg AT, et al. (2014b) Interscalene brachial plexus blocks under general anesthesia in children: is this safe practice? A report from the Pediatric Regional Anesthesia Network (PRAN). *Reg Anesth Pain Med.* 39,502–5.

Varghese E, Deepak KM, Chowdary KV. (2009). Epinephrine test dose in children: is it interpretable on ECG monitor? *Paediatr Anaesth.* 19,1090–5.

Weinberg GL. (2012) Lipid emulsion infusion: resuscitation for local anesthetic and other drug overdose. *Anesthesiology.* 1,180–7.

Weinberg GL, VadeBoncouer T, Ramaraju GA, Garcia-Amaro MF, Cwik MJ. (1998) Pretreatment or resuscitation with a lipid infusion shifts the dose-response to bupivacaine-induced asystole in rats. *Anesthesiology.* 88,1071–5.

Suggested websites

www.aagbi.org/sites/default/files/la_toxicity_2010_0.pdf

www.asra.com/checklist-for-local-anesthetic-toxicity-treatment-1-18-12.pdf

www.sfar.org/article/319/summary [articles in English]

Chapter

5

Basics of ultrasonography for regional anesthesia in children

Christophe Dadure and Chrystelle Sola

Introduction

The use of regional anesthesia in pediatric surgery has been increasing over the last 30 years. Successful neural blockade is essential for good-quality analgesia. Ensuring this can be difficult in pediatric practice, as these techniques can be difficult in younger children due to the close anatomic relationship between nerve and adjacent structures. The use of ultrasound guidance has grown exponentially in recent years in both adults and children. Some blocks that had fallen out of favor, such as the paravertebral and supraclavicular blocks, are increasing as a result of the use of ultrasound. New techniques based on ultrasonography have also appeared. Ultrasound guidance allows visualization of anatomic structures and the accuracy of the local anesthetic (LA) injection. This chapter provides an overview of basic ultrasound technology and equipment use. It will also describe how to identify different structures and some advantages of ultrasound in pediatric regional anesthesia. Ultrasound for specific blocks will be discussed in the relevant block chapters.

Basic principles of ultrasonography

The ultrasound or sonographic image is based on mechanical oscillations of a quartz crystal excited by electrical pulses (piezoelectric effect). Ultrasound probes contain multiple piezoelectric crystals, which are interconnected electronically and vibrate in response to an applied electric current. An ultrasound beam is a continuous or intermittent train of waves emitted by a transducer or probe. These vibrating mechanical sound waves create alternating areas of compression and refraction when propagating through body tissues. Ultrasound waves are characterized by their frequency (measured in cycles per second or hertz), their wavelength (measured in

meters), and their velocity (speed of wave through a medium) (Marhofer, 2011).

The wavelength and frequency of ultrasound are inversely related, i.e. ultrasound of high frequency has a short wavelength and vice versa. Ultrasound frequencies are always higher than 20 000 Hz, which is the upper limit for audible human hearing. Medical ultrasound devices use sound waves in the range of 1–20 MHz. Proper selection of transducer frequency is an important concept for providing optimal image resolution in diagnostic and procedural ultrasound.

As ultrasound waves travel through tissues, they are partly transmitted to deeper structures, partially reflected back as echoes by the different anatomic structures to the transducer, partially scattered, and partially transformed to heat. For imaging purposes, we are mostly interested in the echoes reflected back to the transducer. The amount of echo returned after striking a tissue interface is determined by a tissue property called acoustic impedance. This is an intrinsic physical property of a medium defined as the density of the medium times the velocity of ultrasound wave propagation in the medium. Air-containing organs (such as the lung) have the lowest acoustic impedance, while dense organs such as bone have very high-acoustic impedance. The speed of sound varies in function in different media (Marhofer, 2011).

Different ultrasound modes can be chosen, but for regional anesthesia, B-mode is the optimum mode to use. In B-mode, the echo intensity is represented as different grayscale values. The two-dimensional (2-D) B-mode technique produces a 2-D image in the direction of the sound cone with 50 or more pictures per second, allowing an image in real-time. The M-mode, mainly used in cardiology, is the most basic form of ultrasound imaging. It is generated when the one-dimensional B-mode is recorded over a time bar and

Ultrasound-Guided Regional Anesthesia in Children, ed. Mannion et al. Published by Cambridge University Press.
© Cambridge University Press 2015.

offers the highest time resolution. This mode is useful for the precise timing of events within the cardiac cycle and is often used in combination with color-flow. Color-flow mapping, or "color Doppler," permits mapping and display of blood flow within vessels as different colors and in real-time, while also imaging the static tissues by the 2-D technique. This mode can be used to locate a catheter tip when there is rapid injection of LA through a catheter.

Ultrasound probes, needles, and techniques

Choice of ultrasound probes and needles

High frequency ultrasound waves (short wavelength) generate images of high axial resolution. High frequency waves are more attenuated than lower frequency waves for a given distance; thus, they are mainly suitable for imaging superficial structures. Conversely, low frequency waves (long wavelength) offer images of lower resolution but can penetrate to deeper structures, because of a lower degree of attenuation. The useful frequency for ultrasound-guided peripheral nerve blocks varies between 5 and 15 MHz. It is best to use high frequency transducers (10–15 MHz range) to image superficial structures and low frequency transducers (2–5 MHz) for imaging deeper or neuraxial structures, particularly in adults and larger children. However, for the majority of pediatric practice, a high frequency probe is recommend as neuronal structures are superficial in most children.

Ultrasound probes are named after the geometric arrangement of their piezoelectric elements. We usually distinguish two types of probes (Figure 5.1a):

1. *Curved array probe*: The sound waves are emitted from a single point and diverge fan-wise. This type of probe, with a low frequency (typically 2–5 MHz), is useful for deep structures.

2. *Linear array probes*: The piezoelectric elements are arranged in parallel. They can be activated singly or in groups. The resulting image is square, with good resolution in the near field but with a shallower depth. Linear probes with a high frequency (from 8 to 20 MHz) allow one to perform most regional techniques in children. Linear ultrasound probes exist with a 38 mm or a 25 mm active surface length, which may also be "hockey-stick" shaped (Figure 5.1b).

In principle, the typical needles used to perform peripheral nerve blocks can also be used for ultrasound guidance. In-vitro results have shown that visualization of the needle depends on its diameter and the angle of penetration (Schafhater-Zoppoth et al., 2004). Today, some manufacturers have developed a new generation of needles adapted for ultrasound use. These needles are covered with "cornerstone" reflectors providing an optimal visibility of the needle tip (Figure 5.2).

Technique of puncture

The first step in ultrasound-guided nerve blocks is to visualize all the anatomic structures in the target area. Two techniques of puncture can be performed depending on the needle position relative to the probe:

(a)

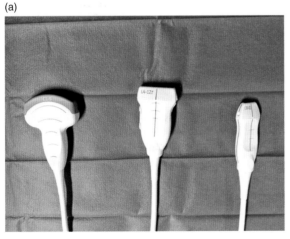

(b)

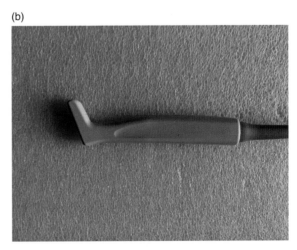

Figure 5.1 Different types of probes. (a) Curve array probe (left), linear array probe 38 mm (middle), and linear array probe 25 mm (right). (b) "Hockey-stick" type probe.

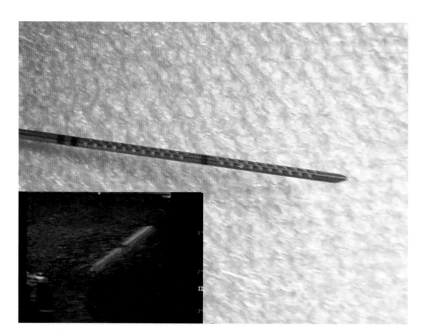

Figure 5.2 Specific needle covered with "cornerstone" reflectors providing optimal sonographic visibility of the tip.

1. *The out-of-plane technique*: The needle is inserted perpendicular to the long axis of the probe. The needle then appears as a hyperechoic dot if the angulation of the needle does not exceed 45 degrees to the wave front (Figure 5.3). Introducing the needle too close to the probe will make it more difficult to see the tip. The needle position can also be identified by tissue movement and displacement, by a dorsal acoustic shadow emerging distal to the tip, or by injection of a small volume of saline or LA. Small translation movements of the probe can also determine the location of the needle tip. The difficulty in this approach is that one is trying to locate the needle tip only, and not the whole needle.

2. *The in-plane technique*: The needle is aligned to the long axis of the probe, allowing the visualization of the needle shaft and tip (Figure 5.4). This technique, while allowing more of the needle to be seen, can still be difficult because it requires that the needle be directly in the ultrasound beam. The probe orientation is very important because small deviations of the probe from the needle path will remove the needle from the screen image. As the probe is typically positioned perpendicular to the nerve, therefore the needle is advanced perpendicular to the long axis of the nerve. This approach may be safer because it allows one to track the progress of the needle (and the tip) in real-time.

It is important to note that, regardless of the approach taken, the trajectory of the needle can be completely different from those customarily used in the nerve stimulation, blind, or "pop" techniques.

Identification of structures in ultrasonography
Neural structures

Nowadays, with the improved resolution of modern ultrasound machines and their associated software, the majority of peripheral nerves for regional anesthesia can be visualized in children. These images are not static and can alter depending on the position of the child, the pressure of the probe on the skin, the progression of the needle, or the injection of LA. Neuronal structures can be imaged transversally (axially) or longitudinally (Figure 5.5). Most imaging is done with the probe scanning the cross-section of the nerve (perpendicular to the long axis of the nerve), allowing the identification of the target nerve, evaluation of its depth, and finding the optimal angle of the probe for maximum echogenicity from the nerve. This change of echogenicity depending on which angle of inclination the transducer is at, is termed anisotropy.

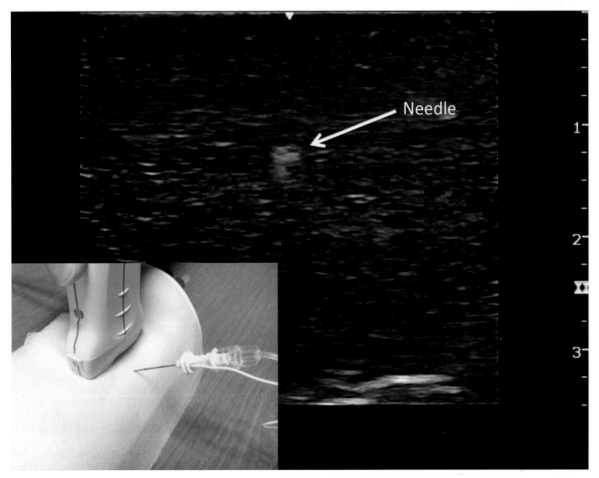

Needle

Figure 5.3 Visualization of the tip of the needle with out-of-plane technique (performed in phantom).

Adjusting for a number of variables on the ultrasound machine can optimize the view of neural structures. These include depth, gain, and frequency and will vary depending on the nerve to be located. Each ultrasound machine is different in terms of how to adjust these settings. The common term is "knobology," and we recommend that the relevant ultrasound machine company provide training before use.

Peripheral nerves may have a hypoechoic (dark structure) or hyperechoic (bright structure) sonographic appearance, depending on the size of the nerve, the sonographic frequency, and the angle of the ultrasound beam. The proximal part of a plexus usually appears hypoechoic, while distal portions are hyperechoic. It is possible to identify the internal structure of a nerve with high frequency transducers. The hypoechoic structures are the fascicles of the nerves while the hyperechoic background reflects the connective tissue between neuronal structures. It is important to note that each nerve has a particular appearance in ultrasonography with regard to its shape and echogenicity. The nerve may also take various shapes (round, oval, or triangular) according to its anatomic location and the surrounding tissues.

Visualization of neural structures is age dependant, particularly of the spinal region. In children, nerve and vascular structures are naturally smaller, at more superficial depths, and usually there is less adipose tissue or muscle septae. In infants less than 1 year of age, the spine and associated structures are readily imaged, but this clarity rapidly decreases as ossification of the vertebral column increases with age. Contrary to the "loss of resistance" technique, the main structure to identify is not the ligament flavum but the dura mater to measure depth.

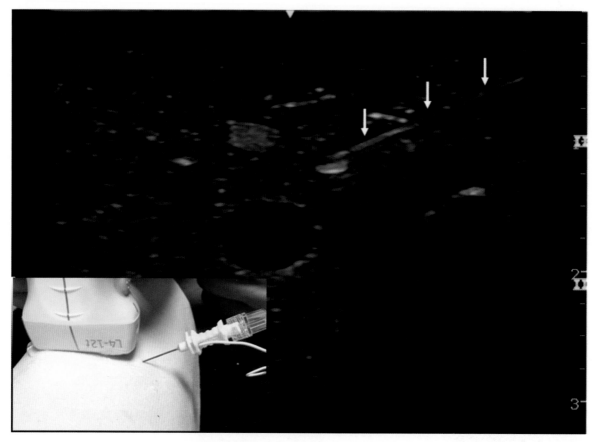

Figure 5.4 Visualization of the needle with in-plane technique (performed in phantom).

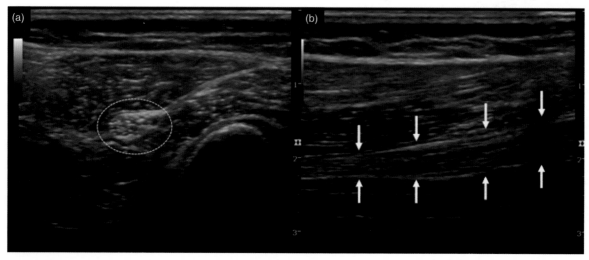

Figure 5.5 Visualization of hyperechoic sciatic nerve structure in a 6-year-old child on (a) transversal approach or (b) longitudinal approach.

Neuraxial structures can be visualized using a longitudinal or transverse approach.

Adjacent structures

In ultrasound guidance, the ability to identify adjacent structures is crucial to avoid any confusion with the neural structures:

- *Bones*: The cortex of bone is hyperechoic and appears as a white line on the ultrasound image. The ultrasound beam being totally reflected, a distal shadow (completely anechoic) is located behind this white line of bone cortex (Figure 5.6).
- *Vessels*: The vessels are identified as round or oval anechoic shape. Their appearance may vary depending on the pressure exerted by the probe, particularly for veins which are easily compressible. Discrimination between arteries and veins is possible with color Doppler (Figure 5.7). It is important to identify the vessels during ultrasound-guided regional anesthesia in order to avoid intravascular injection.
- *Tendons*: During ultrasound-guided regional anesthesia, tendons can cause the most confusion because they have a very similar sonographic appearance to nerves. To distinguish between both, it is important to track them over a short distance. Tendons disappear while the nerves remain visible over these distances.
- *Muscles*: Muscles have a fibrolamellar sonographic appearance. Muscles may appear as either heterogeneous structures with hyperechoic intramuscular septae or homogenous structures (Figure 5.6). Some muscles or their septae are important as they allow easier identification of the target nerve or the space for injection of LA (transversus abdominis plane block or ilioinguinal/iliohypogastric block).
- *Lymph nodes*: These appear as oval or round shapes with a hyperechoic vascular hilus entering

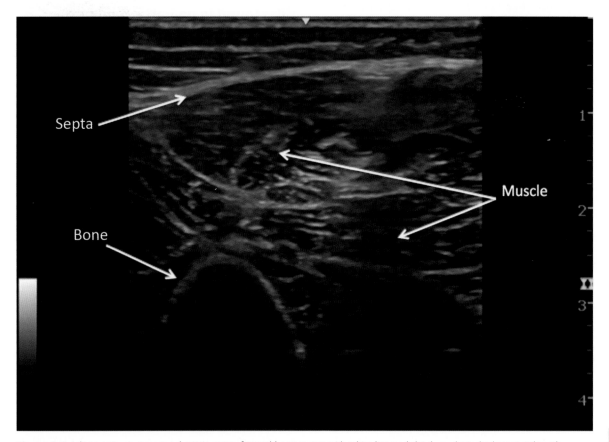

Figure 5.6 Adjacent structures around sciatic nerve: femoral bone cortex with white line and distal anechoic shadow, muscle with fibrolamellar sonographic appearance, and hyperechoic septae.

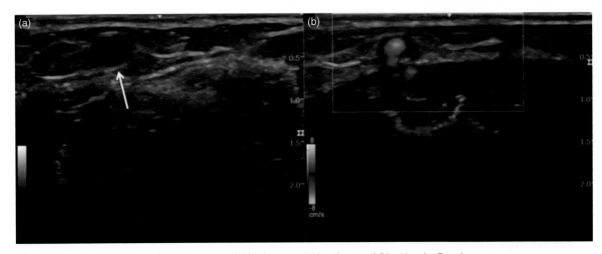

Figure 5.7 Sonographic image of vein in a young child (white arrow) (a) without and (b) with color Doppler.

the lymph node. Color Doppler can help to distinguish it from blood vessels.

- *Air*: This is hyperechoic artefact with distal shadows. Injection of air is sometimes used to locate the catheter tip during regional anesthesia.
- *Local anesthetic*: LA appears as an anechoic puddle in ultrasonography (Figure 5.8). Nerves are often more visible when they are surrounded by LA.

Detailed anatomic knowledge is an absolute pre-requisite for the performance of ultrasonography for regional anesthesia. This knowledge provides the foundation on which to build the operator's under-standing of the sonoanatomy they image and to appreciate anatomic variations. There are a number of well-recognized international workshops teaching cadaveric anatomy for regional anesthesia.

Sterility of procedure

The procedure of ultrasound-guided regional anes-thesia must be performed in a sterile condition. Sterile preparation of the transducer and the block area is an important prerequisite before regional anesthesia. A sterile probe cover must be used for single and continuous blocks procedures. The ultrasound gel used between the probe and the skin of the patient must be sterile. It may also be necessary to put gel between the probe and the protective cover. It does not need to be sterile as it is not in direct contact with the skin.

There are pre-prepared sterile kits including ultrasound gel and a protective cover specifically designed by a number of manufacturers for ultrasound-guided procedures.

Ultrasound in pediatric regional anesthesia

The advantages of the use of ultrasound in regional anesthesia are primarily the real-time visualization of the anatomy of the patient, the precise positioning of the needle, and the direct visualization of LA spread.

In a recent review of literature, other advantages for ultrasound-guided regional anesthesia in children include (Tsui and Pillay 2010):

For ultrasound-guided peripheral nerve blocks (PNBs):

- Faster onset time for upper extremity blocks.
- Improved intraoperative block success rates for truncal PNBs.
- Reduction of volume of LA needed for successful perioperative analgesia.
- The detection of anatomic variants.
- More comfortable block performance in awake children.

By contrast, ultrasound-guided blocks were not being performed faster than conventional localization tech-niques, nor did ultrasound guidance improve success rates in upper extremity PNB in comparison with nerve stimulation techniques.

For ultrasound-guided neuraxial blocks:

- Ultrasonographic guidance allows visualization of the spine and associated structures (ligament

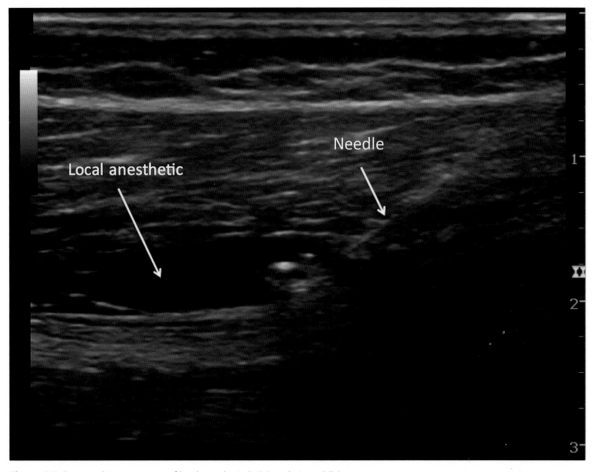

Figure 5.8 Sonographic appearance of local anesthetic (LA) (anechoic puddle).

flavum, dura mater, conus medullaris and cerebrospinal fluid), especially in infants less than 1 year of age.

- Pre-procedural ultrasound imaging offers a moderate prediction of the depth of skin to the epidural space.
- Ultrasound permits visibility of needle within epidural space in neonates.
- Ultrasound guidance can detect catheters during advancement in some young infants; and can confirm epidural catheter placement due to the injection of fluid.
- Reduction of bone contact in infants and children.
- Ultrasounds permit the evaluation of the anatomy of caudal epidural space, especially the relationship of the sacral hiatus to the dural sac and the presence of occult spinal dysraphism.

Ultrasound-guided caudal blocks are superior to the "swoosh" test in terms of sensitivity (96.3% vs. 57.5%, $P < 0.001$) and negative predictive values (40% vs. 5.6%, $P < 0.05$) of caudal epidural placement (Raghunathan et al., 2008). Anterior displacement of the posterior dura mater during saline or LA injection is a predictor of block success. Unfortunately, the image quality is rapidly altered with the ossification of the vertebral column occurring in older children (Marhofer et al., 2005).

Relatively simple ultrasound-guided blocks are axillary blocks, femoral blocks, fascia iliaca compartment blocks, caudal blocks, ilioinguinal blocks, transversus abdominis plane blocks, and rectus sheath blocks. These blocks are suitable for resident teaching and permit a safe and easy learning curve. A comparative evaluation of feasibility with ultrasound guidance versus conventional regional techniques is provided in Table 5.1.

Table 5.1 Evaluation of ultrasound guidance versus conventional techniques of regional anesthesia in children

Technique	Ease to perform conventional techniques	Benefit/risk ratio of US vs. conventional	Feasibility with ultrasound
Central blocks			
Spinal block	Easy	Medium	Moderate
Cervical epidural anesthesia	Avoid	Very low	Avoid
Thoracic epidural anesthesia	Difficult	Medium	Difficult
Lumbar epidural anesthesia	Moderate	Medium	Difficult
Sacral epidural anesthesia	Moderate	Low	Difficult
Caudal block	Easy	High	Easy
Peripheral nerve limbs blocks			
Interscalene block	Moderate	Low	Moderate
Parascalene block	Moderate	Medium	Moderate
Subclavicular block	Moderate	Medium	Moderate
Axillary block	Easy	High	Easy
Psoas compartment block	Difficult	Low	Difficult
Femoral block	Easy	High	Easy
Proximal sciatic blocks	Moderate	Medium	Moderate
Subgluteal sciatic block	Moderate	High	Easy
Popliteal sciatic block	Moderate	High	Easy
Distal block	Moderate	Medium	Difficult
Truncal compartment blocks			
Thoracic paravertebral block	Moderate	Low	Difficult
Rectus sheath block	Easy	Medium	Easy
Ilioinguinal/iliohypogastric nerve block	Moderate	Medium	Easy
Trans abdominis plane block	Easy	Medium	Easy
Penile block	Easy	High	Moderate
Pudendal nerve block	Moderate	Medium	Moderate
Facial and head block			
Trigeminal superficial block	Moderate	High	Moderate
Suprazygomatic maxillary nerve block	Moderate	Medium	Easy
Mandibular nerve block	Easy	Medium	Difficult
Superficial cervical block	Easy	High	Moderate
Occipital nerve block	Easy	Low	Moderate

Ultrasound-guided blocks may become cost-effective techniques, despite the significant upfront costs of an ultrasound machine. A study comparing ultrasound-guided infraclavicular brachial plexus block in comparison to nerve stimulation found that costs were reduced by more than $125 per case taking into account both direct and indirect costs (Sandhu et al., 2004). The major component of these savings was a reduction in onset time that substantially reduced operating room times. Similarly, another study has recently concluded that similar cost reductions are found using ultrasound-guided interscalene block instead of general anesthesia in adult arthroscopic shoulder surgery (Gonano et al., 2009).

Suggested reading

Gonano C, Kettner SC, Ernstbrunner M, et al. (2009) Comparison of economical aspects of interscalene brachial plexus blockade and general anaesthesia for arthroscopic shoulder surgery. *Br J Anaesth.* 103:428–33.

Kriss VM, Desai NS. (1998) Occult spinal dysraphism in neonates: assessment of high-risk cutaneous stigmata on sonography. *Am J Roentgenol.* 171:1687–92.

Marhofer P. (2011) Regional anaesthesia: principles of

localization using ultrasound techniques. In Bissonnette B, ed. *Pediatric Anesthesia: Basic principles – State of Art - Future.* Shelton, CT: People's Medical Publishing House.

Marhofer P, Bosenberg A, Sitzwohl C, et al. (2005) Pilot study of neuroaxial imaging by ultrasound in infants and children. *Paediatr Anesth.* 15:671–6.

Raghunathan K, Schwartz D, Connelly NR. (2008) Determining the accuracy of caudal needle placement in children: a comparison of the swoosh test and ultrasonography. *Paediatr Anesth.* 18:606–12.

Sandhu NS, Sidhu DS, Capan LM. (2004) The cost comparison of infraclavicular brachial plexus block by nerve stimulator and ultrasound guidance. *Anesth Analg.* 98:267–8.

Schafhater-Zoppoth I, McCulloch CE, Gray AT. (2004) Ultrasound visibility of needles used for regional nerve block: an in vitro study. *Reg Anesth Pain Med.* 29:480–8.

Tsui BCH, Pillay JJ. (2010) Evidence-based medicine: assessment of ultrasound imaging for regional anaesthesia in infants, children, and adolescents. *Reg Anesth Pain Med.* 32:S47–54.

Anatomy of the neuraxis, thoracic and abdominal walls, upper and lower limbs

Judith Barbaro-Brown and Gabriella Iohom

Introduction

Ultrasonography is a tool that allows us to visualize with increasing detail internal anatomy such as nerves, vessels, and organs. It can be tempting to use this technology to bypass traditional anatomy learning and to simply identify individual structures in a two-dimensional image. Excellence in regional anesthesia requires intimate and detailed knowledge of the anatomy of the nerves, their neighboring structures, and, most importantly, the functional anatomy of the skin, muscles, or bones these nerves supply. This chapter provides that detail and the background knowledge to perform safe and successful regional anesthesia in children. The Appendix contains a list of tables where the innervation, origin, insertion, and action of each muscle are described – these tables are referenced in the text to their relevant anatomic section.

Neuraxis

The back provides a protective pathway through which the spinal cord passes and spinal nerves exit. The bony contribution is provided by the vertebrae. Ligaments provide supportive connections between the bony elements, and related muscles connect the vertebrae to each other and to adjacent structures, such as the ribs.

Vertebrae

There is a basic structure to all vertebrae with differences occurring depending on their position within the vertebral column. The five categories are:

- Cervical – small in size, foramen situated in transverse processes.
- Thoracic – have articulations for ribs.
- Lumbar – large-sized vertebral bodies. over-lapping articular processes.

- Sacral – five fused vertebrae, with four sacral foramina, and the sacral hiatus.
- Coccygeal – between three and five vertebrae, that may or may not be fused.

A typical vertebra has a vertebral body lying anteriorly to a vertebral arch, the largest vertebral bodies being found in the lumbar area. Each vertebra is separated from its neighbor by a fibro-cartilaginous intervertebral disc.

The vertebral arch is formed posterior to the vertebral body by the two pedicles providing the lateral walls, and the roof formed by the two laminae, joining at the midline. Together these structures surround the vertebral foramen, and the foramina of each vertebra are aligned to form a continuous canal from the magnum foramen in the skull to the lowest point on the sacrum at the sacral hiatus. Within this protective space are the spinal cord and associated membranes, blood vessels, supportive connective tissues, and the emerging spinal nerves.

Along the length of the vertebral column the spinous processes and laminae of adjacent vertebrae partially overlap, forming the transverse foramina through which spinal nerves exit the vertebral canal. In the lumbar region these foramina are relatively wide, and can provide access to the vertebral canal (Figure 6.1).

Spinal cord

The spinal cord lies protected within the vertebral canal, encased in three layers of connective tissue structures known as meninges. The layer closest to the spinal cord is the delicate pia mater, attached directly to the spinal cord. Surrounding this is the arachnoid mater, which does not adhere to the pia mater, creating a space between the two, the subarachnoid space, filled with cerebrospinal fluid.

Ultrasound-Guided Regional Anesthesia in Children, ed. Mannion et al. Published by Cambridge University Press.
© Cambridge University Press 2015.

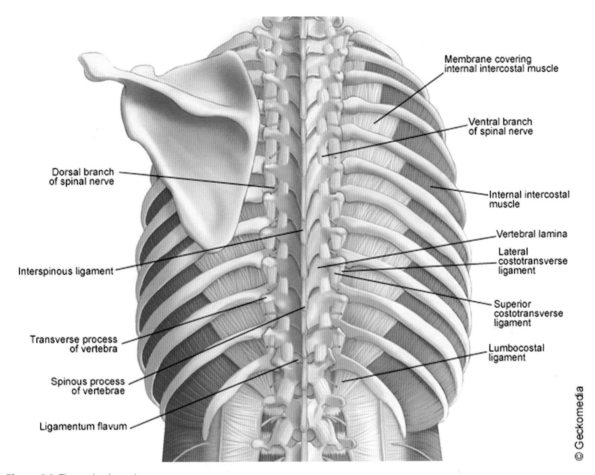

Figure 6.1 Thoracolumbar spine.

The outermost layer is the dura mater, which lies against the arachnoid mater but has no attachment to it. The dura mater does not touch the bony vertebral canal, but is cushioned by fat and connective tissue, and is accompanied within this epidural space by a venous plexus.

The spinal cord passes through the magnum foramen and extends distally to between L1 and L2 (in the adult), although there can be variation between T12 and L3. During childhood development and growth, the vertebral column and spinal cord do not grow at the same speed, with the vertebral column extending at a faster rate, and, therefore, the distal end of the spinal cord appears to be more proximal in the vertebral canal in the adult compared to neonates where it extends to approximately L3 or L4. The spinal cord stops growing between the ages of 4 and 5 years; therefore, the tip of the spinal cord will appear progressively more proximal with continued skeletal growth until this ceases approximately between 16 and 18 years, at which point the spinal cord tip will approximate the level of L2. The terminal point of the spinal cord is cone-shaped (conus medullaris), and a connective tissue filament (the filum terminale) extends from this to anchor at the coccyx. The spinal cord has two large swellings along its length, corresponding to the areas associated with upper and lower limb spinal nerve emergence. The cervical enlargement corresponds to the regions where C5–T1 spinal nerves emerge, whilst the lumbosacral enlargement corresponds to the regions of L1 to S3 spinal nerve emergence.

Spinal nerves

Thirty-one pairs of spinal nerves arise from the spinal cord and emerge from the vertebral canal via the transverse foramina. There are 8 pairs of cervical nerves, 12 pairs of the thoracic region, 5 pairs of the lumbar region, 5 sacral pairs, and

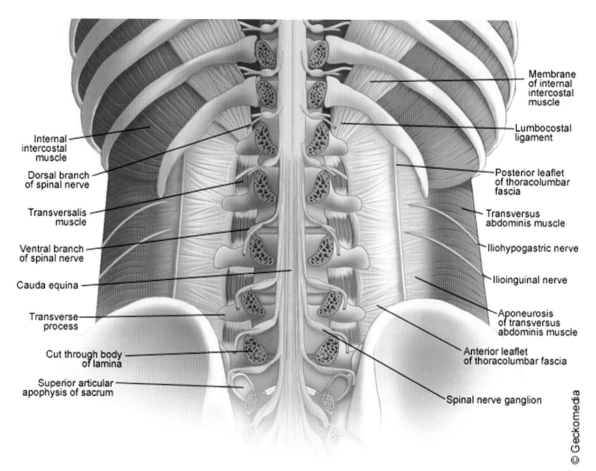

Internal intercostal muscle

Dorsal branch of spinal nerve

Transversalis muscle

Ventral branch of spinal nerve

Cauda equina

Transverse process

Cut through body of lamina

Superior articular apophysis of sacrum

Membrane of internal intercostal muscle

Lumbocostal ligament

Posterior leaflet of thoracolumbar fascia

Transversus abdominis muscle

Iliohypogastric nerve

Ilioinguinal nerve

Aponeurosis of transversus abdominis muscle

Anterior leaflet of thoracolumbar fascia

Spinal nerve ganglion

© Geckomedia

Figure 6.2 Cauda equine.

1 single coccygeal pair. They all arise from the spinal cord as anterior and posterior bundles of rootlets, uniting to form the single spinal nerve before passing through the transverse foramen. The spinal nerves do not always arise at the same level from which they exit the vertebral canal, and distal pairs of spinal nerves (especially those of the lumbar and sacral regions) travel some distance within meningeal membranes inside the vertebral canal before they exit. These "free" spinal nerves at the second to fifth lumbar levels, all sacral levels, and the coccygeal level, form the cauda equina, although the pairs of nerves continue to exit the vertebral canal (Figure 6.2). After this point, each spinal nerve splits into an anterior and posterior branch (anterior and posterior rami). The anterior ramus is the larger branch, and provides innervation of the majority of the body (except the head) whereas the smaller posterior ramus innervates the back.

Ligaments

Ligaments connect adjacent vertebral bodies at a number of points as well as connecting transverse processes and laminae. The major ligaments are:

- Anterior and posterior longitudinal ligaments
- Ligamenta flava
- Ligamentum nuchae
- Supraspinous ligament
- Interspinous ligaments.

Anterior and posterior longitudinal ligaments

These ligaments extend vertically along the anterior and posterior borders of the vertebral bodies. The anterior longitudinal ligament runs from the base of the skull to the anterior surface of the sacrum, joining the anterior aspects of the vertebral discs as well as the vertebral bodies. The posterior longitudinal ligament lies within the vertebral canal, attached to the posterior aspect of the vertebral bodies and discs. It begins at C2, where it is known as the tectorial membrane of the atlanto-axial joint, connecting this vertebra to the base of the skull.

Ligamenta flava

Ligamenta flava occur between the laminae of neighboring vertebrae, preventing separation of the laminae during flexion, whilst helping to maintain back position. They pass obliquely from the anterior surface of the superior lamina to the posterior surface of the inferior lamina.

Thoracic wall

The thoracic wall consists of thoracic vertebrae, intervertebral discs, ribs, sternum, and all the surrounding and interosseous musculature. The thoracic wall extends from the superior thoracic aperture at the level of the first rib and the upper border of the manubrium, to the inferior thoracic aperture at the border of the twelfth rib, the tip of the eleventh rib, the costal margin, and the distal point of the xiphoid process. At the posterior midline, the bodies of the thoracic vertebrae make up the posterior aspect of the thoracic wall.

Skeletal contribution

Thoracic vertebrae articulate with the 12 pairs of ribs posteriorly, whilst anteriorly the first 7 pairs of ribs articulate with the sternum. The next three pairs of ribs articulate anteriorly with the costal cartilages of the rib directly superior, whilst the final two pairs have no anterior articulation.

Between the ribs are the intercostal spaces in which are sited intercostal muscles as well as vessels and intercostal nerves. These latter structures run along the costal groove on the inferior border of each rib, usually with the vein most superior and closest to the rib, inferior to which is the artery, and inferior to the artery is the nerve, which on occasions is completely out-with the costal groove and, therefore, more at risk of damage. Directly overlying the intercostal spaces are muscles contributing to arm movement (Pectoralis major and minor, Subclavius), and superficial to these are the deep fascia, superficial fascia, and skin. Beneath the intercostal spaces and ribs lies the endothoracic fascia, separating the thoracic wall from the underlying pleura.

Muscular components

The roles of the muscles of the thoracic wall are to change rib and sternal position during breathing to create changes in thoracic volume and, therefore, thoracic pressures. The muscles of the thoracic wall are:

- Levatores costarum
- Serratus posterior superior and Serratus posterior inferior
- Intercostals – external, internal, innermost
- Subcostales
- Scalenes
- Transversus thoracis.

Levatores costarum

There are 12 pairs of these small muscles, arising from the tips of the transverse processes of C7–T11. The muscles pass inferolaterally to insert into the rib directly inferior to the vertebra from which they have arisen. They do not play a role in the inspiratory process but contribute to vertebral movement.

Serratus posterior superior and Serratus posterior inferior

Serratus posterior superior arises collectively from the lower border of ligamentum nuchae, the spinous processes of C7, T1–T3, and the supraspinous ligament. It passes inferolaterally and inserts into the upper borders of the second to fifth ribs. The muscle acts to elevate the second to fifth ribs during inspiration. Serratus posterior inferior arises collectively from the spinous processes of T11–L2 and the supraspinous ligament. It passes superolaterally to insert into the inferior borders of the ninth to twelfth ribs. It functions to pull the lower ribs down and backwards to aid in forced expiration, as well as contribution to trunk movement.

Intercostal muscles

These are made up of three elements within each intercostal space, known as (superficial to deep) external, internal, and innermost intercostals. Together they provide support for the ribs during breathing, as well as contribution to rib movement.

External intercostal muscles –– there are 11 pairs of these muscles, each arising from the inferior border of ribs 1–11 and extending to the superior border of the rib directly below (ribs 2–12), running obliquely forwards and downwards. They are active during inspiration and elevate the ribs, widening the rib cage, and increase the dimensions of the thoracic cavity.

Internal intercostal muscles –– the 11 pairs of these muscles arise from the inferolateral edge of the costal grooves of ribs 1–11 and extend to the superior margins of ribs 2–12, deep to the external intercostal muscles. The Internal intercostal muscles also run obliquely, but in the opposite direction to the external layer, i.e. posteroinferiorly, and are active during expiration.

Innermost intercostal muscles –– these muscles arise from the anterior surfaces of the costal grooves and pass directly to the inner surface of the rib directly inferior, running in the same direction as the Internal intercostals. The neurovascular bundles, which run in the costal grooves, lie between the Internal and Innermost intercostal muscles.

Subcostales

This group of muscles runs in the same direction as the Internal intercostals, passing across multiple ribs. They arise from the internal surfaces of the rib, passing medioinferiorly across the rib immediately below before inserting into the internal surface of the rib directly below that, i.e. they span three ribs. These muscles are thought to work in combination with the Internal intercostals during forced expiration.

Scalenes

The scalene muscle group consists of three pairs of muscles – Scalenus anterior, Scalenus medius, and Scalenus posterior. They arise from the transverse processes of C2–C7, with the anterior and medial pair inserting into the superior surface of the first rib, Scalenus medius inserting posteriorly in relation to Scalenus anterior. Scalenus posterior inserts into the superior surface of the second rib, just anterior to the angle of the rib. The anterior and medial Scalenes lift the first rib (as well as contributing to neck flexion), whilst the posterior Scalene raises the second rib (whilst allowing the neck to laterally flex). In addition, they can act as accessory muscles for inspiration. The Scalenes are important clinically because the subclavian artery and the brachial plexus both pass between the anterior and medial Scalenes (the scalene fissure, scalene hiatus). The subclavian vein and the phrenic nerve pass across the anterior aspect of Scalenus anterior where it inserts into the first rib.

Transversus thoracis

These muscles are found on the innermost surface of the anterior thoracic wall, arising from the posterior aspect of the xiphoid process, the lower third of the body of the sternum, and the costal cartilages of ribs 4–7. They run superolaterally to insert into the inferior edges of the costal cartilages of ribs 3–6, lying in the same plan as the Internal intercostal muscles, although there is variation in this insertion between individuals, as well as on opposite sides of the sternum in the same individual. The internal thoracic vessels lie between the Transversus thoracis muscles and the Internal intercostal muscles.

Vascular supply

The thoracic wall is mainly supplied by the anterior and posterior intercostal arteries, running within the intercostal spaces in the costal grooves of the ribs. The intercostal arteries arise from the aorta and internal thoracic arteries. The internal thoracic arteries (internal mammary arteries) arise from the subclavian artery and run down the lateral borders of the body of the sternum together with the internal thoracic vein between the Internal intercostal and the Transversus thoracis muscle layers. The internal thoracic arteries give off two branches at each rib level, the superior branch running along the inferior surface of the upper rib whilst the lower branch anastomoses with a collateral branch from the posterior intercostal artery. The internal thoracic artery then bifurcates near the sixth intercostal space to form the musculophrenic and superior epigastric arteries.

There are 11 paired posterior intercostal arteries that supply the posterior aspect of the intercostal spaces. The first and second branches arise from the supreme intercostal artery, which itself runs down into the thorax as a branch of the costocervical trunk (a posterior branch of the subclavian artery). The third to ninth branches arise from the posterior aspect of the thoracic aorta, but it should be noted that due to the position of the aorta to the left of the vertebral column the posterior intercostal arteries for the right side of the posterior thoracic wall must pass across the vertebral bodies, posterior to the esophagus, thoracic duct, and the azygos vein. The posterior intercostal arteries then run along the inferior border of the corresponding rib, together with the posterior intercostal vein and the intercostal nerve relative to that intercostal space. Further branches arise from the posterior intercostal arteries which anastomose with branches of the anterior intercostal arteries.

The venous system mirrors the arterial supply, with the intercostal veins draining into internal thoracic veins, in turn draining into brachiocephalic veins.

Innervation

Intercostal nerves provide innervation for the thoracic wall, and these are formed from the anterior rami of spinal nerves T1–T11. Spinal nerves exit the dural sleeve at the intervertebral foramen and travel through the paravertebral space to enter the intercostal space becoming intercostal nerves. The intercostal nerves run together with the artery and vein along the lower border of the ribs. The first two intercostal nerves (from T1 and T2) innervate the upper limb in addition to the thoracic wall, the nerves from T3–T6 innervate the thoracic wall only, whilst those from T7–T11 innervate both the thoracic and abdominal walls. The xiphoid process indicates the termination of the seventh intercostal nerve, whilst the umbilicus indicates the termination of the tenth intercostal nerve. The nerve from T12 innervates the abdominal wall and groin.

Abdominal wall

The margins of the abdominal wall are the xiphoid process and costal margins superiorly, the vertebral column posteriorly, and the upper borders of the pelvis inferiorly. There are multiple layers to the abdominal wall consisting of fascia, muscles, peritoneum, and skin.

Superficial fascia

The superficial fascia consists mainly of fatty connective tissue continuous with the superficial fascia of the rest of the body, although anteriorly it forms two layers in the lower region below the umbilicus, referred to as the deeper membranous layer and the superficial fatty layer. The superficial fatty layer, as the name suggests, contains a high proportion of fat and may vary considerably in thickness. It runs over the inguinal ligament and is continuous with the superficial fascia of the thigh. In the male the superficial layer also continues over the penis, and fuses with the deeper layer of superficial fascia over the scrotum, forming the dartos fascia, a specialized layer, which contains smooth muscle, but has low levels of fatty

tissue. In females the levels of fatty tissue remain, and this layer contributes to the labia majora.

The deeper membranous layer is much thinner with lower levels of fat. Inferior to the inguinal ligament it fuses with the fascia lata in the thigh, whilst in the midline of the abdomen it blends with the linea alba and the symphysis pubis. Inferiorly it runs into the perineum and attaches to the inferior pubic ramus (ischiopubic ramus) and the posterior aspect of the perineal membrane, sometimes referred to as Colles' fascia. In the male the deep and superficial fascial layers blend to form the superficial fascia of the penis, subsequently contributing to the dartos fascia. Extensions of the deeper layer also attach to the pubic symphysis of the male to form the fundiform ligament of the penis. In females the deeper layer extends into the labia majora and the anterior aspect of the perineum.

Muscles

The five muscles of the abdominal wall are sited antero-laterally and are described as either flat or vertical:

- Flat – External oblique, Internal oblique, Transversus abdominis
- Vertical – Rectus abdominis, Pyramidalis.

The flat muscles arise posterolaterally and run forwards towards the midline, gradually being replaced by aponeurosis at the midline, whereas the vertical muscles run within the aponeurosis arising from the flat muscles, and are situated para-laterally to the midline. Together these muscles work synergistically as a support mechanism for the abdominal organs to maintain them within the abdominal cavity, and also to maintain posture.

Transversus abdominis –– this is the deepest of the three flat muscles, lying under the internal oblique muscle. It blends with the linea alba at the midline.

Internal oblique –– this is the intermediate muscle of the flat muscle group. It is a relatively small and thin structure when compared to the External oblique muscle. This muscle also blends at the midline with the linea alba, and its fibers run superomedially.

External oblique –– this is the most superficial of this muscle group, and lies immediately below the superficial fascia. Its fibers run inferomedially, and as it blends with the other muscles in the group it contributes a large aponeurotic component to the anterior aspect of the wall. From the inferior border of the aponeurosis of the External oblique muscle the inguinal ligament arises, running from the anterior superior iliac spine anteroinferiorly to attach to the pubic tubercle. The inguinal ligament also forms part of the inguinal canal. At the anterior end of the inguinal ligament there are a number of other ligaments formed: the lacunar ligament arises as a crescent-shaped structure, which runs backwards to insert into the pecten pubis on the iliopubic ramus, and further elements arise from the lacunar ligament at this point to form the pectineal ligament (Cooper's ligament).

All three flat muscles are each surrounded by a layer of deep fascia, the layer specifically related to the Transversus abdominis muscle being known as the transversalis fascia. This layer is continuous with the lining of the abdominal and pelvic cavities, as well as the fascial layer on the inferior aspect of the diaphragm, and the deep fascia of the muscles on the posterior abdominal wall and the thoracolumbar fascia.

Rectus abdominis -- this is a flat, paired muscle separated by the linea alba in the midline. It runs from the costal margin to the pubic symphysis, being wider and thinner superiorly. In those with well-developed Rectus muscles it is possible to see transverse fibrous banding at intervals along the length of the muscle.

Pyramidalis -- as the name would suggest, Pyramidalis is triangular in shape, and may not be present in all individuals. The base of the triangle arises from the pubis with the apex inserting into the linea alba, the muscle belly lying anterior to Rectus abdominis.

Both vertical muscles are also enclosed in a structure known as the rectus sheath consisting of the aponeuroses of the Internal and External obliques, and the Transversus abdominis muscles. The lower quarter posterior surface of the Rectus abdominis muscle is not covered by the rectus sheath, and, therefore, is in immediate contact with the transversalis fascia at this point.

Extraperitoneal fascia

Deep to the transversalis fascia is the extraperitoneal fascia, separating it from the peritoneum. The extraperitoneal fascia lines the abdominal cavity and is continuous with the lining of the peritoneal cavity. The fascia is thicker and fattier on the posterior aspect of the abdominal wall (forming the pararenal fascia around the kidneys), but becoming thinner and more fibrous towards the linea alba. Beneath the extraperitoneal fascia lies the peritoneum, which is a thin, serous membrane providing the innermost layer of the abdominal wall (parietal peritoneum). In some areas this reflects onto the abdominal organs to provide either a partial or complete covering (visceral peritoneum). In females, the parietal peritoneum forms a sac with small openings allowing the uterine tubes to pass through. In males this sac is closed, but in both cases this sac forms the peritoneal cavity.

Vascular supply

The arterial supply (mirrored by venous drainage) of the abdominal wall can be considered in superficial and deep layers.

Superficial layer -- superiorly, it is supplied by branches of the musculophrenic artery (arising from the internal thoracic artery), whilst the inferior aspect of the wall is supplied laterally by the superficial circumflex iliac artery, and medially by the superficial epigastric artery, both of which arise from the femoral artery.

Deep layer -- the superior aspect of the deep supply is from the superior epigastric artery (a terminal branch of the internal thoracic artery), whilst the deep lateral aspect arises from the tenth and eleventh intercostal arteries together with the subcostal artery. Inferiorly the supply is from the inferior epigastric artery and deep circumflex iliac artery, both of which arise from the external iliac artery. Both the inferior and superior epigastric arteries run posterior to Rectus abdominis, eventually anastomosing with each other.

Innervation

The spinal nerves of T7--T12 and L1 provide innervation to the anterolateral parietal peritoneum, muscles, and skin, passing from posterior to anterior and giving off smaller lateral cutaneous branches (Figure 6.3). The intercostal nerves of T7--T11 run deep to the costal cartilage and run forward to the anterolateral wall between Transversus abdominis and the Internal oblique muscle. They pass posteriorly to the lateral border of the rectus sheath and give off an anterior cutaneous branch, which passes through Rectus abdominis to the skin. Eventually all

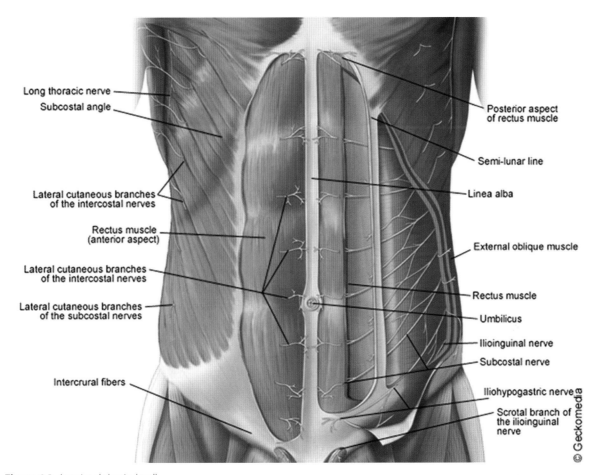

Long thoracic nerve

Subcostal angle

Lateral cutaneous branches of the intercostal nerves

Rectus muscle (anterior aspect)

Lateral cutaneous branches of the intercostal nerves

Lateral cutaneous branches of the subcostal nerves

Intercrural fibers

Posterior aspect of rectus muscle

Semi-lunar line

Linea alba

External oblique muscle

Rectus muscle

Umbilicus

Ilioinguinal nerve

Subcostal nerve

Iliohypogastric nerve

Scrotal branch of the ilioinguinal nerve

© Geckomedia

Figure 6.3 Anterior abdominal wall.

these nerves provide cutaneous supply, with T7–T9 innervating the skin from the xiphoid process to the umbilicus; T10 supplying the skin of the umbilicus; T11, T12, and L1 innervating the area inferior to the umbilicus to the pubic region. L1 also provides a branch known as the ilio-inguinal nerve, which innervates the anterior surface of the labia majora/scrotum, with a small cutaneous branch running to the thigh.

Upper limb

The upper limb consists of the shoulder, arm, forearm, and hand. A number of areas represent important structural landmarks and indicate transitions between differing components of the upper limb, i.e. the axilla, cubital fossa, and the carpal tunnel, through which major vessels and nerves will pass. For the purposes of this book, the anatomy of the bones, muscles and vessels below the elbow will not be discussed.

The *axilla* is a triangular-shaped area formed by the muscles and bones of the shoulder together with the lateral aspect of the thoracic wall. The boundaries consist of the posterior axillary fold and anterior axillary fold. Latissimus dorsi and Teres major form the posterior axillary fold, whilst the inferior border of Pectoralis major forms the anterior axillary fold. Within the axilla run the axillary artery and vein, a portion of the brachial plexus, lymph nodes, and the long thoracic nerve and intercostobrachial nerve.

Bones

The bones of the arm include the scapula and clavicle, which articulate with the proximal end of the humerus as the glenohumeral joint. At its distal end the humerus articulates with the radius and ulna at the elbow to allow flexion and extension.

Muscles

Shoulder region

The muscles in the shoulder region attach to the humerus, scapula, and clavicle. There are two muscle groups in this region, which lie deep and superficial. The Trapezius and Deltoid, with Levator scapulae and Rhomboid major and minor lying directly beneath, form the superficial group (Appendix table A.1). Deep to all these muscles are Supraspinatus, Infraspinatus, Teres minor, and Teres major, all sited posteriorly. A number of these muscles contribute to the rotator cuff, a musculo-tendinous structure that contributes to shoulder stability (Supraspinatus, Infraspinatus, Teres minor, Subscapularis). The deep group of muscles passes between the scapula and the proximal aspect of the humerus, along with the long head of Triceps brachii (Appendix table A.2).

Arm

The arm describes the region from the shoulder joint to the elbow joint, and consists of two muscular compartments separated by the medial and lateral intermuscular septa, running from the humerus to the deep fascia (Appendix table A.3). Anteriorly are the muscles that flex the elbow – Coracobrachialis, Brachialis, and Biceps brachii – all commonly innervated by the musculocutaneous nerve. Posteriorly there is only one extensor muscle – Triceps brachii, innervated by the radial nerve. As the names suggest for Biceps brachii and Triceps brachii, these muscles have more than one point of origin. The three heads of Tricep brachii eventually converge to form a common insertion into the olecranon process.

Vascular supply

The upper limb is supplied by the subclavian artery, which gives off a number of branches to the head, neck, and chest as well as scapular branches before becoming the axillary artery at the level of the first rib. The axillary artery supplies the walls of the axilla and related regions, and is divided into three parts by Pectoralis minor which crosses the vessel: part 1, proximal to the muscle; part 2, posterior to the muscles; and part 3, distal to the muscle, with six branches arising from these parts:

- Part 1 – superior thoracic artery
- Part 2 – thoracoacromial artery, lateral thoracic artery
- Part 3 – subscapular artery, anterior humeral circumflex artery, posterior circumflex humeral artery.

The axillary artery runs laterally to the axillary vein, and the artery is surrounded by the brachial plexus. Part 2 of the axillary artery provides a reference point for the cords of the brachial plexus, the posterior cord so-called because it lies deep to part 2 of the axillary artery, which itself lies posterior to Pectoralis minor.

The axillary artery then passes across the distal aspect of Teres major, after which it becomes known as brachial artery. The brachial artery runs down the ventral aspect of the arm, and gives off a number of branches:

- Profunda brachii artery (deep brachial artery)
- Superior ulnar collateral artery
- Inferior ulnar collateral artery
- Nutrient branches to the humerus.

The median nerve runs close to the brachial artery, lying immediately lateral to it in the proximal region but moving medially in the distal region, before lying anterior to the brachial artery at the elbow. As the artery reaches the cubital fossa, it divides into the radial and ulnar arteries, which go on to supply the forearm.

The arterial system in the upper limb is mirrored by an accompanying venous network, with an interconnected system of deep and superficial vessels. The superficial vessels form a plexus which drains into the deeper vessels, themselves running with the arteries.

There are two major veins – the cephalic and basilic veins. The cephalic vein arises from the lateral side of the dorsal venous network, and runs up the arm superficially to pass between Pectoralis major and the Deltoid muscle before passing into the axilla where it drains into the axillary vein. The basilic vein arises from the medial side of the dorsal venous network. At the cubital fossa there can be a connection between the basilic and cephalic veins (the medial cubital vein), before the basilic vein continues proximally on the medial aspect of the biceps muscle, and at the lower border of Teres major joins with the anterior and posterior circumflex humeral veins, after which it drains into the brachial veins to form the axillary vein.

Innervation

Innervation of the upper limb arises from the brachial plexus formed from the anterior rami of the spinal nerves of C5–C8, and an anterior ramus of T1. The brachial plexus originates in the neck before passing inferolaterally over the first rib and into the axilla. The brachial plexus is divided into roots, trunks, divisions, and cords, the latter of which provide the major nerves for the upper limb. The proximal sections of the brachial plexus lie posterior to the subclavian artery in the neck, whilst the distal sections surround the axillary artery.

Roots and trunks

Roots arise directly from the anterior rami of C5–C8, and T1, with C5 and C6 becoming the superior trunk, C7 providing the middle trunk, and C8 and T1 providing the inferior trunk (Figure 6.4). The roots and trunks enter the posterior triangle of the neck between the anterior and middle scalene muscles, lying superior and posterior to the subclavian artery. The trunks run laterally across the first rib and enter the axilla.

The superior and middle trunks are superior to the subclavian artery whilst the inferior trunk is posterior to the artery at this point.

Divisions

The three trunks divide further, each producing a posterior and an anterior division. The anterior divisions eventually give rise to peripheral nerves supplying the anterior muscle compartments of the arm and forearm, whereas the posterior divisions supply the posterior compartments, although no peripheral nerves arise directly from these divisions.

Cords

There are three cords (Figures 6.5 and 6.6).

- Lateral – formed by the anterior divisions of the superior and middle trunks, and lies laterally to part 2 of the axillary artery.

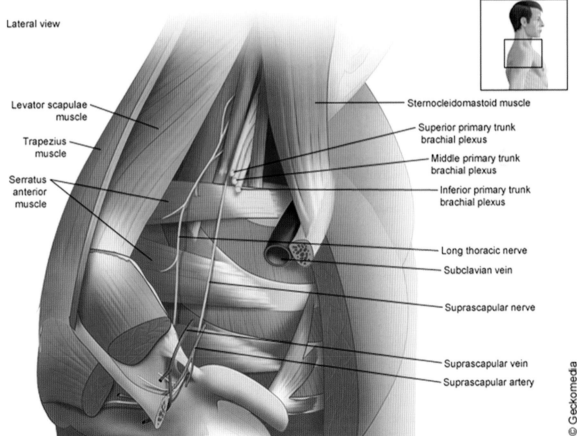

Lateral view

Levator scapulae muscle

Trapezius muscle

Serratus anterior muscle

Sternocleidomastoid muscle

Superior primary trunk brachial plexus

Middle primary trunk brachial plexus

Inferior primary trunk brachial plexus

Long thoracic nerve

Subclavian vein

Suprascapular nerve

Suprascapular vein

Suprascapular artery

© Geckomedia

Figure 6.4 Trunks of the brachial plexus.

49

Anterior view

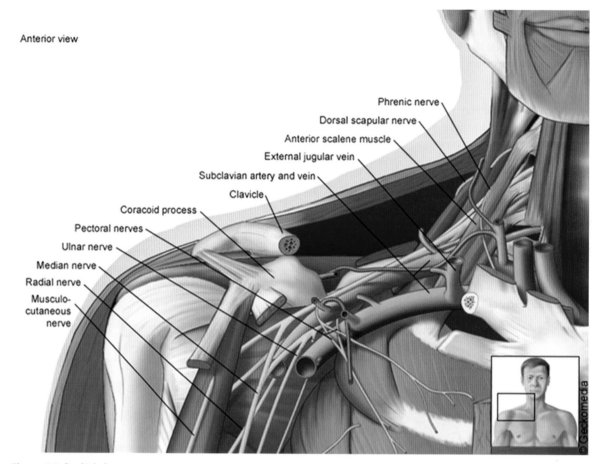

Phrenic nerve
Dorsal scapular nerve
Anterior scalene muscle
External jugular vein
Subclavian artery and vein
Clavicle
Coracoid process
Pectoral nerves
Ulnar nerve
Median nerve
Radial nerve
Musculo-
cutaneous
nerve

Figure 6.5 Brachial plexus.

- Posterior – formed by all three posterior divisions, lying posteriorly to part 2 of the axillary artery.
- Medial – the continuation of the anterior division of the inferior trunk, and lies medial to part 2 of the axillary artery.

The lateral and medial cords provide innervation for anterior compartments, and the posterior cord innervates posterior compartments. All motor innervation in the upper limb is provided by one of the five terminal nerves of the brachial plexus (Figure 6.7).

Terminal nerves

Axillary nerve (C5, C6)

The axillary nerve (posterior cord) arises at the level of the axilla, supplying the Deltoid, Teres minor, and the long head of Triceps brachii, as well as sensory innervation to the skin over the inferior region of the Deltoid. It initially runs posterior to the axillary artery

but anterior to Subscapularis, running inferiorly to the muscle's lower aspect. It then follows the path of the posterior humeral circumflex artery, through a quadrilateral space formed by Teres major and Teres minor, the long head of Triceps brachii, and the surgical neck of the humerus, after which it splits into anterior, posterior, and a number of collateral branches (Figure 6.8):

- The anterior branch runs around the surgical neck of the humerus, beneath the Deltoid together with the posterior humeral circumflex vessels. This branch also provides a number of small cutaneous branches which supply the overlying skin.
- The posterior branch supplies Teres minor and the posterior part of the Deltoid. The branch then passes through the deep fascia and continues as the superior lateral cutaneous nerve of arm, running around the posterior aspect of the Deltoid and supplying the skin over the inferior

Anterior view

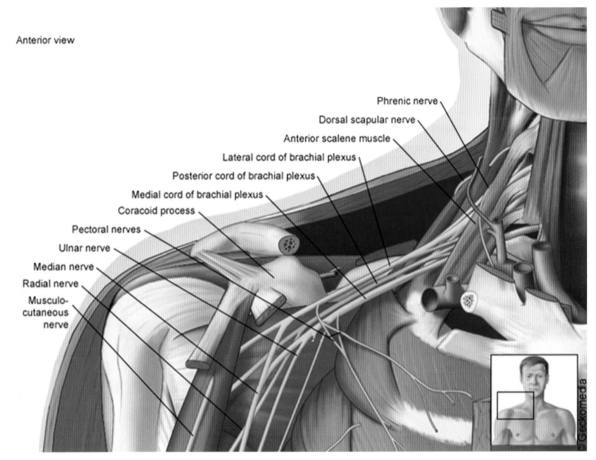

Phrenic nerve
Dorsal scapular nerve
Anterior scalene muscle
Lateral cord of brachial plexus
Posterior cord of brachial plexus
Medial cord of brachial plexus
Coracoid process
Pectoral nerves
Ulnar nerve
Median nerve
Radial nerve
Musculo-
cutaneous
nerve

Figure 6.6 Brachial plexus with the vessels removed.

two-thirds of the posterior part of this muscle, as well as the skin overlying the long head of Triceps brachii.

Musculocutaneous nerve (C5, C6, C7)

The musculocutaneous nerve (lateral cord) arises from the brachial plexus at the level of the lower border of Pectoralis major. It passes through Coraco-brachialis before running obliquely between Biceps brachii and Brachialis, towards the lateral aspect of the arm. Superior to the elbow it passes through the deep fascia lateral to the tendon of Biceps brachii and continues as the lateral cutaneous nerve of the fore-arm. During its course as the musculocutaneous nerve it innervates Coracobrachialis, Biceps brachii, and Brachialis. However, there can be variations to the course of the nerve, and in some cases it runs medially rather than laterally and passes beneath Biceps brachii rather than through Coracobrachialis.

Median nerve (C5, C6, C7, C8, T1)

The median nerve originates from the medial and lateral cords of the brachial plexus, and is the only nerve to pass through the carpal tunnel at the wrist. Once it arises from the brachial plexus it passes out of the axilla and into the arm at the lower border of Teres major before running inferiorly together with the brachial artery. Its path is between Biceps brachii and Brachialis, but at first it runs lateral to the brachial artery before moving anteriorly to the vessel, subsequently running medially to the artery in the cubital fossa. Here it runs anterior to the insertion of Brachialis, and deep to Biceps brachii. As it runs across the elbow joint, the median nerve gives off an articular branch.

After leaving the cubital fossa and entering the forearm, the median nerve passes between the heads of Pronator teres and travels inferiorly between Flexor digitorum profundus and Flexor digitorum superficialis. The nerve innervates the anterior muscle

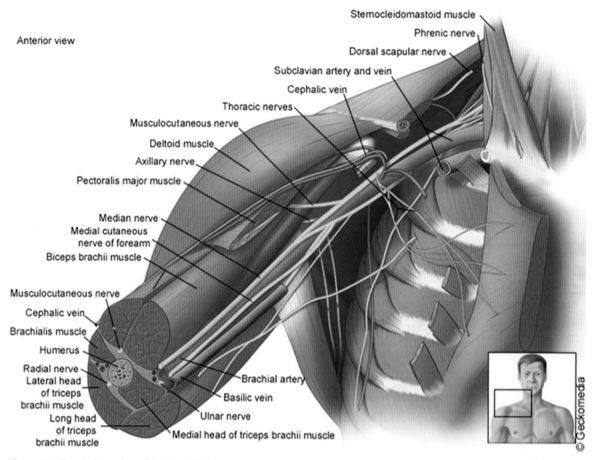

Anterior view

Sternocleidomastoid muscle
Phrenic nerve
Dorsal scapular nerve
Subclavian artery and vein
Cephalic vein
Thoracic nerves
Musculocutaneous nerve
Deltoid muscle
Axillary nerve
Pectoralis major muscle
Median nerve
Medial cutaneous nerve of forearm
Biceps brachii muscle
Musculocutaneous nerve
Cephalic vein
Brachialis muscle
Humerus
Radial nerve
Lateral head of triceps brachii muscle
Long head of triceps brachii muscle
Brachial artery
Basilic vein
Ulnar nerve
Medial head of triceps brachii muscle
© Geckomeda

Figure 6.7 Terminal branches of the brachial plexus.

compartment, specifically the superficial and intermediate muscles, with the exception of Flexor carpi ulnaris. The median nerve finally emerges between Flexor digitorum superficialis and Flexor pollicis longus. During its passage through the forearm the median nerve gives off two branches:

- The anterior interosseous branch, which runs with the anterior interosseous artery, innervating the muscles of the deep anterior compartment of the forearm, with the exception of the medial section of Flexor digitorum profundus and Flexor carpi ulnaris. This branch terminates as it innervates Pronator quadratus.

- The palmar cutaneous branch arises at the distal part of the forearm and provides sensory supply to the lateral aspect of the skin of the palm. The palmar cutaneous branch does not pass through the carpal tunnel, but instead runs in a separate fascial groove next to Flexor carpi radialis and then above the flexor retinaculum.

After passing through the carpal tunnel, the median nerve enters the hand and provides a number of further branches, although in some individuals (between 5 and 10%) this bifurcation may occur within the carpal tunnel or even more proximally in the wrist or forearm. The branches are:

- A recurrent branch to the muscles of the thenar compartment where it provides innervation to Opponens pollicis, Abductor pollicis brevis, and the superficial part of Flexor pollicis brevis.

- A common palmar digital branch and a proper palmar digital branch to supply the lateral 3½ digits on the palmar side and the dorsal aspect of the second to fourth digits.

Ulnar nerve (C8, T1)

The ulnar nerve is the largest "exposed" nerve in the body in that it is protected by neither bone nor muscle, and is, therefore, more liable to direct trauma. It arises from the medial cord of the brachial plexus and runs

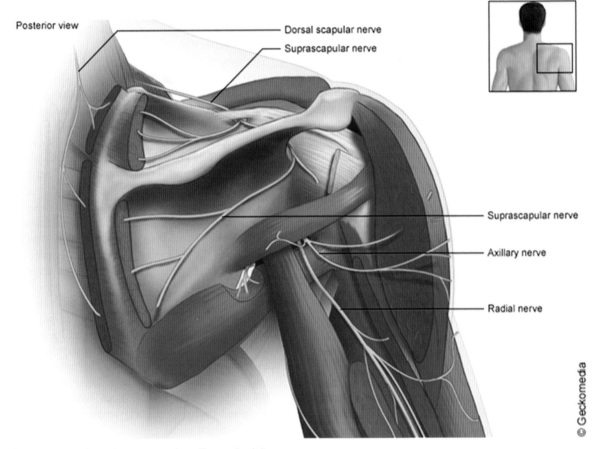

Posterior view

Dorsal scapular nerve

Suprascapular nerve

Suprascapular nerve

Axillary nerve

Radial nerve

© Geckomedia

Figure 6.8 Dorsal scapular, suprascapular, axillary, and radial nerves.

posteromedially to the humerus. It does not supply any structures in the arm, but instead supplies the forearm and hand. It enters the forearm between the heads of the humerus and ulna (sending a branch to the elbow joint), alongside Flexor carpi ulnaris, which it supplies, together with the medial half of Flexor digitorum profundus. The ulnar nerve runs inferiorly with the ulnar artery, and gives off three branches:

- Muscular branches of ulnar nerve – supplies Flexor carpi ulnaris and Flexor digitorum profundus (medial half).
- Palmar branch of ulnar nerve – cutaneous innervation to the anterior skin of the hand and the nails.
- Dorsal branch of ulnar nerve – cutaneous innervation to the posterior skin of the hand, but not the nails.

The ulnar nerve passes into the hand superficial to the flexor retinaculum, through the ulnar canal. At this point a further two branches are given off – the deep and superficial branches of the ulnar nerve:

- Deep branch – supplies the hypothenar muscle group, the third and fourth Lumbricals, the Dorsal and Palmar interossei, Adductor pollicis, and the deep head of Flexor pollicis brevis.
- Superficial branch – supplies Palmaris brevis only.

Sensory innervation is also provided for the fifth digit and the medial half of the fourth digit, together with the related area of the palm.

Radial nerve (C5, C6, C8, T1)

The radial nerve arises from the posterior cord of the brachial plexus, and supplies the Triceps brachii in addition to the extensor compartment of the forearm, the overlying skin on the forearm, and sections of the dorsal aspect of the hand. As it arises from the brachial plexus, it runs in the posterior compartment of the arm with the axillary and brachial artery before

53

moving into the anterior compartment. In the forearm it runs in the posterior compartment. In the arm it gives off a branch to the medial head of Triceps brachii before running through the radial sulcus in the humerus, innervating the lateral head of the Triceps (the long head of the Triceps is innervated by the axillary nerve). The nerve emerges onto the lateral aspect of the humerus and passes through the lateral intermuscular septum to enter the anterior compartment of the arm, where it runs between Brachialis and Brachioradialis. At the distal aspect of the humerus the radial nerve runs in front of the lateral epicondyle and on into the forearm where is provides a number of further branches:

- The superficial branch of the radial nerve passes inferiorly in the forearm underneath Brachioradialis before crossing that muscle to lie in the posterior aspect of the forearm. It supplies sensory innervation to the dorsal aspects of the hand, the first and second digits, and the radial aspect of the third digit, up to the distal interphalangeal joints.
- The deep branch of the radial nerve pierces the Supinator muscle (innervating it) and runs around the radius to the posterior aspect of the forearm. It passes through the Supinator muscle again and becomes known as the posterior interosseous nerve of forearm. It passes through the posterior extensor muscles and runs on the posterior interosseous membrane, just below Extensor pollicis brevis accompanied by the posterior interosseous artery, terminating at the Extensor retinaculum. It supplies Extensor digitorum, Extensor digit minimi, Extensor carpi ulnaris, Extensor carpi radialis brevis, Abductor pollicis longus, Extensor pollicis brevis, Extensor pollicis longus, and Extensor indicis.

Muscular branches of the radial nerve also innervate Triceps brachii, Anconeus, Brachioradialis, and Extensor carpi radialis longus. The radial nerve also provides sensory innervation via the posterior cutaneous nerve of the arm, the inferior lateral cutaneous nerve of the arm, and the posterior cutaneous nerve of the arm.

Collateral nerves around the brachial plexus

- The dorsal scapular nerve (ventral ramus of C5) innervates Rhomboid major and minor, and Levator scapulae. The nerve passes through Scalenus medius and runs deep to the Rhomboids and Levator scapulae, together with the dorsal scapular artery or sometimes the transverse cervical artery (Figure 6.8).
- The long thoracic nerve arises from the anterior rami of C5, C6, and C7, although in some cases the contribution from C7 is absent. The contributions from C5 and C6 pass through Scalenus medius, whilst the contribution from C7 passes anterior to the same muscle. The nerve runs inferiorly posterior to the brachial plexus and axillary artery, and innervates Serratus anterior (Figure 6.4).
- The suprascapular nerve arises from the superior trunk of the brachial plexus, with C5 and C6 as its nerve roots. The nerve runs across the posterior triangle of the neck deep to Trapezius before running along the superior aspect of the scapula (Figure 6.8). It passes inferior to the superior transverse scapular ligament and through the suprascapular notch, entering the supraspinous fossa. It subsequently runs beneath Supraspinatus and around the lateral aspect of the scapular spine, towards the infraspinous fossa. The nerve carries both motor and sensory fibers, innervating Supraspinatus and Infraspinatus, whilst providing sensation to the acromioclavicular and glenohumeral joints.
- The lateral pectoral nerve arises from the lateral cord of the brachial plexus, with nerve roots C5–C8. It runs across the axillary artery, passing through the deep fascia and innervating Pectoralis major. It also communicates with the medial pectoral nerve to form the ansa pectoralis.
- The medial pectoral nerve arises from the medial cord of the brachial plexus, via nerve roots C8 and T1. It runs behind part 1 of the axillary artery and communicates with the lateral pectoral nerve in front of the axillary artery, after which it innervates Pectoralis minor and Pectoralis major.
- The upper subscapular nerve, sometimes known as the superior subscapular nerve, arises from the posterior cord of the brachial plexus derived from C5 and C6. It passes directly into and innervates Subscapularis.
- The thoracodorsal nerve arises from the posterior cord of the brachial plexus, derived from C6, C7, and C8, and is sometimes known as the long subscapular nerve. It runs with the subscapular

artery towards Latissimus dorsi, which it innervates.

- The lower subscapular nerve arises from the posterior cord of the brachial plexus, via nerve roots C5 and C6. It innervates Subscapularis and Teres major.

- The medial brachial cutaneous nerve (or medial cutaneous nerve of the arm) arises from the medial cord of the brachial plexus, from C8 and T1. It is the smallest branch from the brachial plexus and passes through the axilla with the axillary vein, communicating with the intercostobrachial nerve. It runs inferiorly to the middle of the arm, accompanied by the brachial artery, before passing through the deep fascia to supply the skin on the posterior aspect of the lower third of the arm, as far as the elbow. It also communicates with the medial antebrachial cutaneous nerve.

- The medial antebrachial cutaneous nerve (or the medial cutaneous nerve of the forearm) also arises from the medial cord of the brachial plexus, from C8 and T1. As it passes the axilla it provides a small branch, which innervates the skin over Biceps brachii. The nerve runs down the arm medial to the brachial artery, and together with the basilic vein it passes through the deep fascia, subsequently dividing into volar and ulnar branches. The volar branch is the larger of the two, and runs anteriorly down the ulnar aspect of the forearm, innervating the overlying skin as far as the wrist, and communicating with the palmar cutaneous branch of the ulnar nerve. The ulnar branch runs obliquely down the arm medial to the basilic vein before passing anterior to the medial epicondyle of the humerus and into the forearm, where it continues down the ulnar aspect of the forearm to the wrist and innervates the overlying skin. It finally communicates with the dorsal branch of the ulnar nerve, the dorsal antibrachial cutaneous branch of the radial nerve, and the medial brachial cutaneous nerve.

Lower limb

The lower limb is divided into a number of topographic regions – gluteal, thigh, leg, and foot. Other areas have been described from the perspective of structural relationships, and these are the femoral triangle, the popliteal fossa, and to a lesser extent the posteromedial aspect of the ankle. For the purposes of this book, the anatomy of the bones, muscles, and vessels below the knee will not be discussed.

The femoral triangle is situated in the medioproximal aspect of the thigh, the borders of which are the inguinal ligament, the medial borer of Sartorius, and the lateral border of Adductor magnus. The femoral artery, femoral vein, and femoral nerve all pass beneath the inguinal ligament approximately half way along its length, and together these three structures pass downwards to leave the femoral triangle at the apex formed by Sartorius and Adductor magnus.

The popliteal fossa sits behind the knee joint and is a lozenge (or diamond-shaped) structure bordered superiorly by the medial borders of the long head of Biceps femoris, Semimembranosus and Semitendinosus, whilst inferiorly the borders consist of the medial and lateral heads of Gastrocnemius. The popliteal artery and popliteal vein run through the fossa, as does the tibial nerve and the common peroneal nerve (fibular nerve), before running to supply the leg and foot.

Bones

Within the gluteal region is the pelvis (made up by the ilium, ischium, pubis, sacrum, and coccyx), which articulates with the femur at the hip joint. At the distal end the femur articulates with the tibia and the patella, forming the knee joint.

Muscles

Gluteal region

In this region there are two muscle groups, one lying deep to the other. The superficial group is relatively large and is responsible for moving the hip joint and helping to maintain stability and posture (Appendix table A.4). The deep group is relatively small, and mainly contributes to lateral hip rotation (Appendix table A.5). A band of fibrous tissue, known as the fasciae latae, is a deep fascial layer enclosing the thigh, attached proximally to the inguinal ligament and distally to the head of the fibula. On the lateral aspect of the thigh this fascial band thickens, forming the iliotibial band, running from the iliac crest to the lateral condyle of the tibia. Its role is mainly related to stabilization, supported in this by a small muscle – Tensor fasciae latae. This muscle contracts to tighten the iliotibial band when the knee joint is extended, as well as stabilizing the pelvis and minimizing hip adduction.

Some muscles acting on the hip do not originate in the lower limb, but instead extend from the abdominal wall. These are the two muscles that together form the Iliopsoas, and which insert onto the femur (Appendix table A.6).

Thigh

There are a number of muscles in the thigh, which are situated anteriorly (flexing the hip and extending the knee), medially (adducting the thigh), and posteriorly (extending the hip and flexing the knee). The anterior group consists of five muscles, four of which work together as a functional unit referred to as the quadriceps (Rectus femoris and the three Vasti muscles), and Sartorius. The quadriceps muscles all have different origins, but insert jointly into the patella as the patella tendon (Appendix table A.7).

The medial muscle group mainly adducts the thigh (Appendix table A.8). This whole muscle compartment is separated from the anterior compartment by the medial intermuscular septum. There is no similar septum separating them from the posterior muscle group.

Posteriorly, there are three large muscles, sometimes collectively known as the hamstrings, and they are separated from the anterior muscle group by the lateral intermuscular septum (Appendix table A.9). All of these muscles have a common origin, and cross both the hip and knee joints. Biceps femoris inserts laterally onto the fibula, whilst the other two insert medially and can be easily palpated. The sciatic nerve runs vertically through this muscle group, lying deep to the long head of Biceps femoris, where it also branches into the tibial and common peroneal nerves.

Vascular supply

The lower limb is supplied by the femoral artery, a continuation of the external iliac artery as it passes under the inguinal ligament. It usually gives off a branch known as the deep artery of the thigh (profunda femoris), before continuing down the thigh via the adductor canal, medial to the femur. The deep artery of the thigh runs closer to the femur than the femoral artery, and is more posterior, running between Pectineus and Adductor longus. The deep artery of the thigh gives off three main branches:

- The lateral femoral circumflex artery.
- The medial femoral circumflex artery.
- The perforating arteries, which perforate Adductor magnus and run to the posterior and lateral compartments of the thigh.

The femoral artery continues down the thigh in the adductor canal beneath Sartorius before passing through the adductor hiatus within Adductor magnus, to pass to the posterior aspect of the thigh, where it is known as the popliteal artery. This passes between the femoral condyles into the popliteal fossa. The popliteal artery gives off many genicular branches to supply the knee joint and surrounding muscles as well as the sural artery, and it is accompanied on its course by the popliteal vein. As the popliteal artery leaves the popliteal fossa it bifurcates into the anterior and posterior tibial arteries, although in some individuals this bifurcation can occur more proximally and within the popliteal fossa.

Venous return in the foot, leg, and thigh mirrors the distribution of the arterial supply, with the deep veins in the foot eventually joining to form the veins, which run with the main arteries throughout the limb. In addition to this deep venous system, superficial veins drain into the dorsal venous arch, eventually forming the great and small saphenous veins.

The great saphenous vein is the largest of the superficial veins, and runs over the medial malleolus, the medial aspect of the leg, and the medial epicondyle of the femur, before passing through the saphenous opening in the fasciae latae to join the femoral vein.

The small saphenous vein is very superficial and runs with the sural nerve. It passes between the heads of Gastrocnemius and joins with the popliteal vein.

Innervation

Innervation in the lower limb arises from the lumbar and sacral plexuses on the posterior abdominal and pelvic walls. These plexuses are formed by the anterior rami of L1–L3 and most of L4 (lumbar plexus) and L4–S5 (sacral plexus) (Figure 6.9).

Lateral femoral cutaneous nerve -- arises from the dorsal divisions of spinal nerves L2 and L3. It emerges from the lateral border of Psoas major and crosses the Iliacus muscle obliquely, towards the anterior superior iliac spine. It then runs under the inguinal ligament and over Sartorius, into the thigh, where it divides into an anterior and a posterior branch.

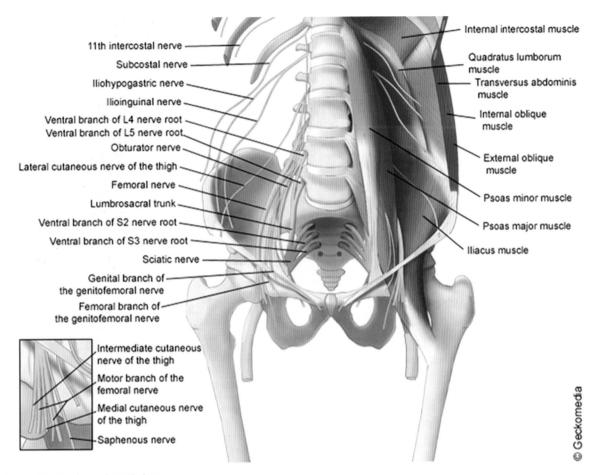

11th intercostal nerve

Subcostal nerve

Iliohypogastric nerve

Ilioinguinal nerve

Ventral branch of L4 nerve root

Ventral branch of L5 nerve root

Obturator nerve

Lateral cutaneous nerve of the thigh

Femoral nerve

Lumbrosacral trunk

Ventral branch of S2 nerve root

Ventral branch of S3 nerve root

Sciatic nerve

Genital branch of the genitofemoral nerve

Femoral branch of the genitofemoral nerve

Intermediate cutaneous nerve of the thigh

Motor branch of the femoral nerve

Medial cutaneous nerve of the thigh

Saphenous nerve

Internal intercostal muscle

Quadratus lumborum muscle

Transversus abdominis muscle

Internal oblique muscle

External oblique muscle

Psoas minor muscle

Psoas major muscle

Iliacus muscle

© Geckomedia

Figure 6.9 Lumbar and sacral plexuses.

The *anterior branch* becomes superficial about 10 cm below the inguinal ligament, and divides into branches, which are distributed to the skin of the anterior and lateral parts of the thigh, extending to the knee. The terminal filaments of this nerve frequently communicate with the anterior cutaneous branches of the femoral nerve, and with the infrapatellar branch of the saphenous nerve, forming the peripatellar plexus.

The *posterior branch* pierces the fascia latae, and subdivides into filaments, which pass backward across the lateral and posterior surfaces of the thigh, supplying the skin from the level of the greater trochanter at the hip, to the middle of the thigh.

Femoral nerve -- the femoral nerve arises from the dorsal divisions of the ventral rami of L2–L4. It descends through Psoas major, emerging from the muscle at the lower part of its lateral border, and passes down between it and Iliacus (Figure 6.10). It continues beneath the inguinal ligament and enters the femoral triangle, where it splits into an anterior and a posterior division, itself providing cutaneous, muscular, and articular branches.

The anterior division gives off anterior cutaneous and muscular branches. The anterior cutaneous branches are the intermediate cutaneous nerve and medial cutaneous nerve. The muscular branches are the nerve to Pectineus, which arises immediately below the inguinal ligament, and passes behind the femoral sheath to enter the anterior surface of the muscle. The nerve to Sartorius arises together with the intermediate cutaneous nerve.

The *posterior division* gives off the saphenous nerve, and muscular and articular branches.

Saphenous nerve -- is the largest cutaneous branch of the femoral nerve (Figure 6.11). It lies in front of the femoral artery and follows the adductor canal

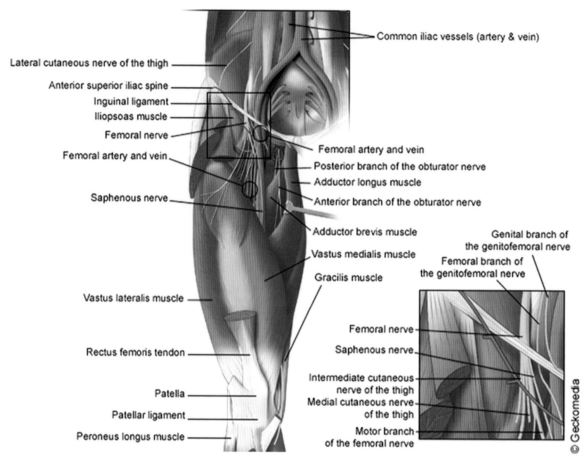

Figure 6.10 Femoral nerve.

(subsartorial canal) as far as the adductor foramen. At this point it leaves the course of the artery and emerges from behind the lower edge of the aponeurotic covering of the canal. It passes directly down along the medial side of the knee, pierces the fascia lata, between the tendons of the sartorius and gracilis, and becomes subcutaneous at this point. It then passes along the tibial side of the leg, accompanied by the great saphenous vein, descends behind the medial border of the tibia, and, at the lower third of the leg, divides into a further two branches. One continues its course along the margin of the tibia, and ends at the ankle, whilst the other passes in front of the ankle, and is distributed to the skin on the medial side of the foot, as far as the first metatarsal phalangeal joint, where it communicates with the medial branch of the superficial peroneal nerve.

Muscular branches –– these supply the four parts of the quadriceps compartment. The branch to Rectus

femoris enters the upper part of the deep surface of the muscle. The branch to Vastus lateralis accompanies the descending branch of the lateral circumflex artery to the lower part of the muscle. The branch to Vastus medialis descends laterally to the femoral vessels together with the saphenous nerve, before it enters the muscle belly. The branches to Vastus intermedius enter the anterior surface of the muscle at mid-thigh level.

Articular branches –– there are three in number to the knee-joint. The first is a long slender filament, derived from the nerve to Vastus lateralis, which penetrates the knee joint capsule of the joint on its anterior aspect. A further branch, derived from the nerve to Vastus medialis, runs downward on the surface of this muscle to near the joint where it penetrates the muscular fibers, and accompanies the articular branch of one of the genicular arteries to supply the synovial membrane. The third branch is derived from the nerve to Vastus intermedius.

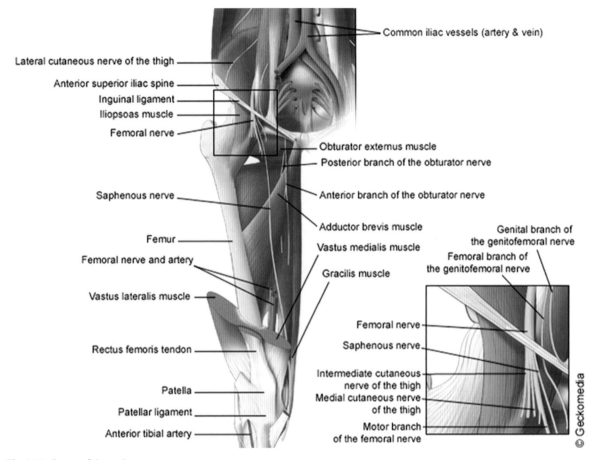

Common iliac vessels (artery & vein)

Lateral cutaneous nerve of the thigh

Anterior superior iliac spine

Inguinal ligament

Iliopsoas muscle

Femoral nerve

Obturator externus muscle

Posterior branch of the obturator nerve

Anterior branch of the obturator nerve

Saphenous nerve

Adductor brevis muscle

Vastus medialis muscle

Femur

Femoral nerve and artery

Gracilis muscle

Genital branch of the genitofemoral nerve

Femoral branch of the genitofemoral nerve

Vastus lateralis muscle

Femoral nerve

Saphenous nerve

Rectus femoris tendon

Intermediate cutaneous nerve of the thigh

Medial cutaneous nerve of the thigh

Patella

Patellar ligament

Motor branch of the femoral nerve

Anterior tibial artery

© Geckomedia

Fig 6.11 Course of the saphenous nerve.

Obturator nerve -- formed from the anterior branches of L2–L4. It descends through the fibers of Psoas major, and emerges from its medial border near the pelvic brim (pelvic aperture). It then passes behind the common iliac vessels, and on the lateral side of the hypogastric vessels and ureter, which separate it from the ureter, and runs along the lateral wall of the lesser pelvis (area below the pelvic brim), above and in front of the obturator vessels, to the upper part of the obturator foramen. It passes through the obturator canal and enters the thigh. Here, it divides into an anterior and a posterior branch. The obturator nerve is responsible for the sensory innervation of the skin of the medial aspect of the thigh. In terms of motor supply, it innervates the adductor muscles – Obturator externus, Adductor longus, Adductor brevis, Adductor magnus, and Gracilis.

Posterior cutaneous nerve of the thigh -- arises from the sacral plexus, partly from the dorsal divisions of

S1 and S2, and from the ventral divisions of S2 and S3. It leaves the pelvis through the greater sciatic foramen below Piriformis, before descending beneath Gluteus maximus with the inferior gluteal artery, and running down the back of the thigh beneath the fasciae latae, and over the long head of the Biceps femoris to the back of the knee (Figure 6.12). At this point it passes through the deep fascia and runs with the short saphenous vein to the middle of the back of the leg, where it communicates with the sural nerve. Its branches are all cutaneous, and are distributed to the gluteal region, the perineum, and the back of the thigh and leg. The main part to the back of the thigh and leg consists of numerous filaments derived from both sides of the nerve, and distributed to the skin covering the back and medial side of the thigh, the popliteal fossa, and the upper part of the back of the leg.

Sciatic nerve -- the sciatic nerve supplies almost all of the skin of the leg, the muscles of the back of the

59

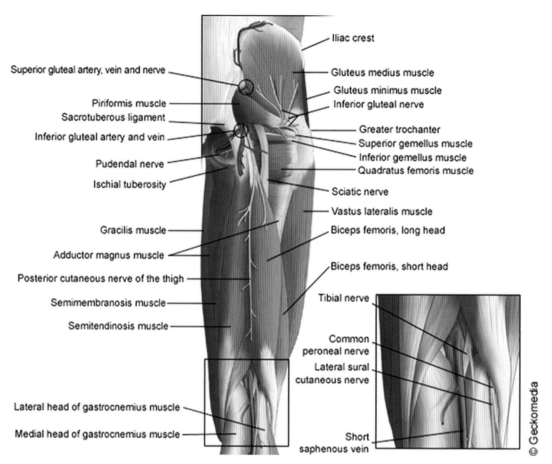

Figure 6.12 Posterior cutaneous nerve of the thigh.

thigh, and those of the leg and foot. It is derived from spinal nerves L4–L5, and S1–S3 and contains fibers from both the anterior and posterior divisions of the lumbosacral plexus, giving off articular and muscular branches, and eventually becoming the tibial nerve.

Articular branches (rami articulares) -- arise from the upper part of the nerve and supply the hip, perforating the posterior part of its capsule; they are sometimes derived from the sacral plexus.

Muscular branches (rami musculares) -- distributed to Biceps femoris, Semitendinosus, Semimembranosus, and Adductor magnus. The nerve to the short head of the Biceps femoris comes from the common peroneal part of the sciatic, whilst the other muscular branches arise from the tibial portion. The muscular branch eventually gives off the tibial nerve and common peroneal nerve, which innervate the muscles of the leg (Figure 6.13). The tibial nerve goes on to

innervate all muscles of the foot except the Extensor digitorum brevis (which is innervated by the peroneal nerve).

Tibial nerve -- the tibial nerve passes through the popliteal fossa to pass below the arch of soleus. In the popliteal fossa the nerve gives off branches to Gastrocnemius, Popliteus, Soleus and Plantaris. Additionally, there are articular branches to the knee joint, and a cutaneous branch, which subsequently becomes the sural nerve. The sural nerve is joined by fibers from the common fibular nerve and runs down the lateral side of the leg to supply the lateral side of the foot. Below Soleus the nerve runs close to the tibia, and supplies the muscles of the deep flexor compartment – Tibialis posterior, Flexor digitorum longus and Flexor hallucis longus. The tibial nerve passes into the foot running behind the medial malleolus, together with the posterior tibial artery, passing under the flexor retinaculum via the tarsal

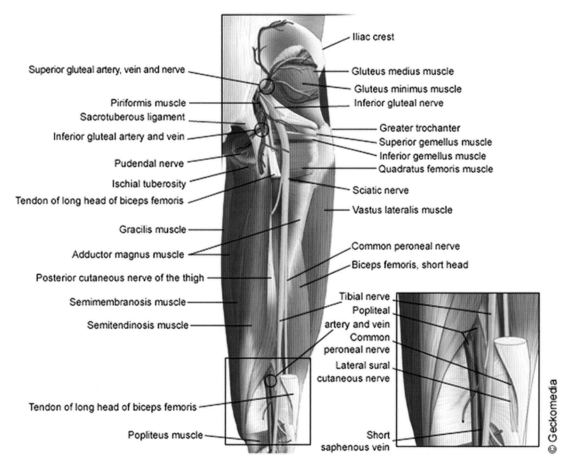

Figure 6.13 High division of the sciatic nerve.

tunnel, where the tibial nerve splits into the medial and lateral plantar nerves.

Medial plantar nerve –– this is the larger of the two terminal divisions of the tibial nerve, and follows the path of the medial plantar artery. It passes under Abductor hallucis and gives off a proper digital plantar nerve before dividing opposite the bases of the metatarsals into three common digital plantar nerves. The branches of the medial plantar nerve are cutaneous, muscular, articular, a proper digital nerve to the medial side of the great toe, and three common digital nerves. The cutaneous branches supply the plantar aspect of the foot; the muscular branches supply Abductor hallucis, Flexor digitorum brevis, Flexor hallucis brevis, and the first Lumbricals.

Lateral plantar nerve –– this is the smaller of the terminal divisions of the tibial nerve, supplying the skin of the fifth digit and lateral half of the fourth, as well

as most of the deep muscles. It runs obliquely forward with the lateral plantar artery to the lateral side of the foot, lying between Flexor digitorum brevis and Quadratus plantae, before dividing into a superficial and a deep branch. Before its division, it supplies Quadratus plantae and Abductor digiti minimi. Afterwards it supplies the skin of the fifth and fourth digits, as the fourth and fifth common digital nerves, themselves giving off cutaneous and articular branches.

Common fibular nerve (common peroneal nerve) –– this is the smaller of the two branches of the sciatic nerve with its original spinal derivation being the dorsal branches of L4–L5 and S1–S2. It runs downward obliquely along the lateral side of the popliteal fossa to the head of the fibula, close to the medial border of Biceps femoris. It lies between the tendon of Biceps femoris and the lateral head of Gastrocnemius, and winds around the neck of the fibula (where it is relatively superficial), between Peroneus longus and the fibula. At this level is gives off articular and lateral sural cutaneous branches, before it divides beneath Peroneus longus into the superficial fibular nerve (superficial peroneal nerve) and deep fibular nerve (deep peroneal nerve).

Articular branches -- there are three articular branches, two of which accompany the superior and inferior lateral genicular arteries to the knee. The third articular nerve is given off at the point of division of the common fibular nerve, and ascends to the front of the knee.

Lateral sural cutaneous nerve -- this supplies the skin on the posterior and lateral surfaces of the leg.

Superficial fibular nerve (superficial peroneal nerve) -- this innervates Peroneus longus and Peroneus brevis, together with the skin over the greater part of the dorsum of the foot (with the exception of the first interdigital space). It passes forward between the peroneal muscles and Extensor digitorum longus, pierces the deep fascia at the lower third of the leg, and finally divides into a medial dorsal cutaneous nerve and an intermediate dorsal cutaneous nerve. As well as this, the nerve gives off muscular branches to the Peroneal muscles, and provides cutaneous filaments to the lower leg.

Deep fibular nerve (deep peroneal nerve) -- this runs between the upper section of the fibula and the upper part of Peroneus longus, passing inferomedially, and deep to Extensor digitorum longus, to the anterior surface of the interosseous membrane. Here it runs with the anterior tibial artery, first lying on the lateral side of the artery, then in front of it, and again on its lateral side at the anklejoint. The nerve and artery descend together to pass anterior to the ankle joint, after which it divides into a lateral and a medial terminal branch. In the leg, the deep fibular nerve supplies muscular branches to Tibialis anterior, Extensor digitorum longus, Peroneus tertius (if present), and Extensor hallucis longus, and an articular branch to the ankle joint.

Acknowledgements

We would like to thank Callimedia, Parc de Bellegarde, Bât A1 Chemin de Borie, F-34170 Castelnau-le-Lez, France for permission to publish the figures contained in this chapter which are from their NATOM Collection © CALLIMEDIA 2014.

Suggested reading

Drake R, Vogl AW, Mitchell WM. (2014) *Gray's Anatomy for Students*, 3rd edn. Philadelphia, PA: Churchill Livingstone.

Moore KL, Agur AMR, Dalley AF. (2014) *Essential Clinical Anatomy*, International edition. Baltimore, MD: Lippincott Williams & Wilkins.

Netter FH. (2014) *Atlas of Human Anatomy*, 6th edn. Philadelphia, PA: Saunders.

Sobotta J, Putz R, Pabst R, Putz R. (2008) *Sobotta Atlas of Human Anatomy: Head, Neck, Upper Limb, Thorax, Abdomen, Pelvis, Lower Limb*, 14th edn. Baltimore, MD: Elsevier Urban and Fischer.

7

Ultrasound-guided axillary brachial plexus block

Pádraig O'Scanaill and Brian O'Donnell

Clinical use

The axillary brachial plexus block (AxBPB) is a commonly performed upper limb block in children, which provides both anesthesia and analgesia for painful upper limb procedures. It is suitable for surgical interventions on the hand, wrist, forearm and elbow. Described by Hirschel in 1911, the AxBPB technique has been modified and incorporated into routine clinical practice. The first report of a successful AxBPB in infants and children appeared in the 1950s (Small, 1951; Fisher et al., 1999).

AxBPB is commonly performed using ultrasound in children following induction of general anesthesia.

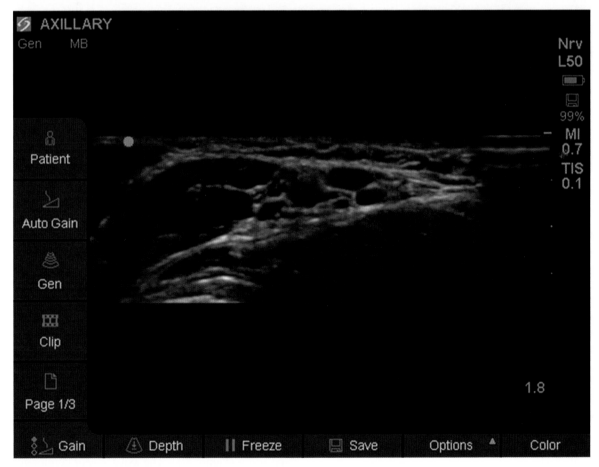

Figure 7.1 Sonoanatomy for axillary brachial plexus block (AxBPB).

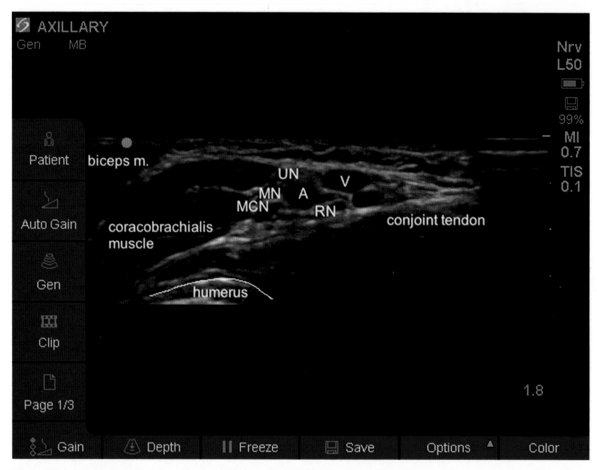

Figure 7.2 Labeled sonoanatomy for axillary brachial plexus block (AxBPB). A, axillary artery; MCN, musculocutaneous nerve; MN, median nerve; RN, radial nerve; UN, ulnar nerve; V, axillary vein.

The distance from skin to plexus is shorter in children than in adults, and the target nerves lie at variable positions around the axillary artery. Given the anatomic location, the absence of structures such as the pleura, phrenic nerve and great vessels, the incidence and magnitude of complications with the ultrasound-guided AxBPB are low compared to other regional techniques (Fisher et al., 1999; Theroux et al., 2007). The use of ultrasound in children has been shown to: (1) lessen the occurrence of block-related complications; (2) reduce the number of needle passes performed during the block procedure; and (3) limit the volume of local anesthetic (LA) used when compared to nerve stimulation alone (McNaught et al. 2011).

The use of ultrasound permits the identification of vessels and the selection of a safe needle path. Avoidance of vessel puncture lessens the risk and occurrence of hematoma formation in AxBPB (Ecoffey et al., 2014).

The use of AxBPB as an adjunct to general anesthesia provides excellent intraoperative and post-operative analgesia. An insensate limb during surgery limits the quantity of both volatile agent and opioid analgesia required (Morton, 2004). Successful AxBPB can hasten transit through the post-anesthesia care unit (PACU) and facilitate early ward or home discharge as a result of improved analgesia and reduced nausea and vomiting.

Clinical sonoanatomy

The anatomy of interest is centered around the axillary artery (Figure 7.1). The axillary vein commonly lies immediately adjacent to the artery however there can be significant variation between individual patients. For descriptive purposes, the position of the nerves

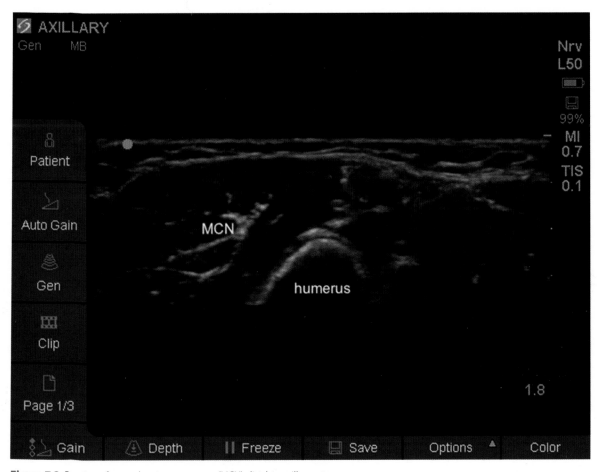

Figure 7.3 Postion of musculocutaneous nerve (MCN) distal to axillary artery.

relative to the axillary artery will be described by referring to clock face terminology (Figure 7.2). The 12 o'clock position faces the skin; the 6 o'clock position faces the humerus and the conjoined tendon of teres major and latissimus dorsi; 9 o'clock faces the coracobrachialis muscle.

The median nerve normally lies close to the axillary artery, usually found between the 9 and 12 o'clock positions. The median nerve has contributions from both the medial and lateral cords and may appear as two distinct entities visible in the axilla.

The ulnar nerve commonly lies between 1 and 4 o'clock in relation to the artery, and commonly sits between axillary artery and vein. Not infrequently the ulnar nerve is in very close relation to the axillary vein, which may envelope the nerve.

The radial nerve may be difficult to visualize; however, in the axilla it lies on the tendon of teres major between 6 o'clock and 4 o'clock on the artery. It is often seen just below the ulnar nerve.

The position of the musculocutaneous nerve is very variable. The musculocutaneous nerve usually leaves the brachial plexus just below the clavicle, and lies in a fascial plane between the coracobrachialis and the biceps muscles (Figure 7.3). Occasionally, the musculocutaneous nerve does not branch off before the axilla, in which case it is still part of the lateral cord and resides close to the median nerve at 9 o'clock on the artery (Figure 7.2).

Variation in the axillary vasculature has been described in the literature with the prevalence of axillary artery variation ranging between 5 and 18% (Cadver et al., 2000). It is thought that axillary artery variability results from abnormal embryonic development of the limb bud vascular plexuses, which is of importance in performing the AxBPB.

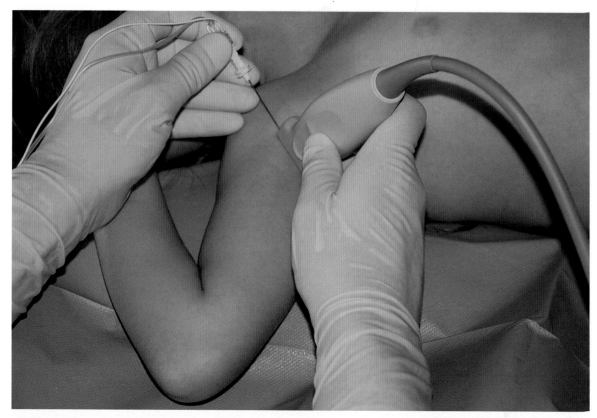

Figure 7.4 Patient position and probe placement. In-plane needle technique.

Innervation of the surgical site in the upper limb may involve more than one component of the brachial plexus. Knowledge of the neural anatomy of the upper limb is imperative for understanding the nerves that need to be blocked. In clinical practice, blocking of all the components of the plexus is recommended because of inter-individual variation and overlap in sensory territories.

Landmarks

With the child in a supine position, the arm is abducted to 90 degrees, the shoulder externally rotated, and the elbow flexed to 90 degrees. The important surface landmarks are: the anterior axillary line medially, the posterior axillary line inferiorly, and the pectoralis major tendon superiorly (Figure 7.4). A high frequency linear ultrasound probe is placed on the skin of the axilla. The ultrasound probe should be oriented to obtain a transverse (axial) view of the underlying structures. Dynamic ultrasound probe movement proximally and distally allows identification of the relevant anatomy. The key structure to identify is the pulsating non-compressible axillary

artery. The nerves can be found around the artery as described above.

Block performance

An in-plane or out-of-plane approach may be adopted utilizing a 22-gauge short bevel needle, usually 25–50 mm depending on the child's size. The majority of clinicians opt for direct needle visualization using the in-plane technique (Chan et al. 2007), as this allows visualization of the needle tip throughout the procedure and of the spread of LA around the target nerves (Figure 7.5).

The choice of LA is dependent on desired onset and duration of block. Lidocaine 2% with epinephrine (1:200 000) has a rapid onset (5–15 min) and duration of approximately 3–4 hours. Bupivacaine/levobupivacaine 0.25% has slower onset (20–30 min) and a duration of 8–10 hours. The dose of LA used for children can be limited by the use of ultrasound (Amiri and Espander, 2010). There are no published data on the recommended LA total dose that should be used for AxBPB in the pediatric population. Common recommended volumes are 0.2–0.3 ml/kg.

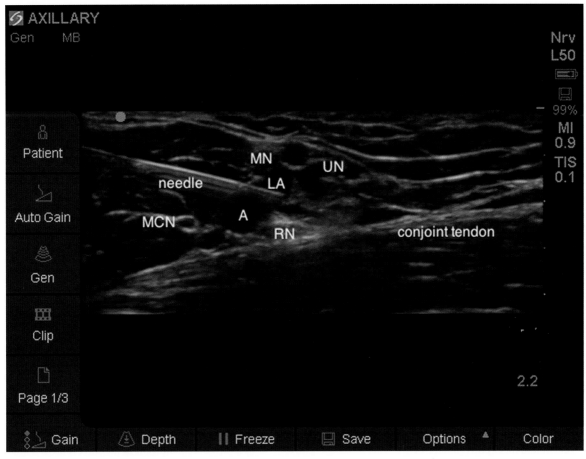

Figure 7.5 Needle insertion and local anesthetic (LA) placement. A, axillary artery; MCN, musculocutaneous nerve; MN, median nerve; RN, radial nerve; UN, ulnar nerve.

The use of very low dose LA in AxBPBs have been described for adult anesthesia (O'Donnell and Iohom, 2009; Ferraro et al., 2014).

Postoperative care

The principles of postoperative care for the AxBPB are similar to other peripheral nerve blocks. Many patients may have a shorter inpatient stay if the appropriate support for patient discharge following regional anesthesia is in place (Wedel et al., 1991). Care of the insensate limb is important, particularly in the pediatric population. Following discharge, an appropriate environment with optimal supervision from parents is required which can reduce risk of injury to the limb. Educating parents on the nature of the AxBPB, expected duration of block, and the importance of meticulous care of the insensate limb until full sensory and motor function has returned is paramount. The affected limb must be placed in a protective sling to avoid injury. Both oral and written information should be provided with details relevant to the block and contact information for the anesthesia team.

Clinical tips

- The axillary brachial plexus block (AxBPB) is easy to perform with ultrasound guidance in the pediatric population.
- There is a very low rate of complications with the AxBPB.
- Ultrasound use in pediatric patients allows direct visualization of anatomic variations of the axillary structures.
- Ultrasound allows direct visualization of the LA perineurally with the possibility of depositing a lower volume.

- The radial nerve lies on the tendon of teres major at 4–6 o'clock, and is often seen below the ulnar nerve, but can be difficult to see.

- The musculocutaneous nerve may lie discrete from the plexus in the plane between the coracobrachialis and the biceps muscles or can be found close to the median nerve at 9 o'clock.

Suggested reading

Amiri HA, Espander R. (2010) Upper extremity surgery in younger children under ultrasound-guided supraclavicular brachial plexus block: a case series. *J Child Orthop.* 4(4),315–19.

Cadver A, Zeybek A, Bayramicli M. (2000) Rare variation of the axillary artery. *Clin Anat.* 13,66–8.

Chan VWS, Perlas A, McCartney CJL, et al. (2007) Ultrasounds guidance improves success rate of axillary brachial plexus block. *Can J Anaesth.* 54(3),176–82.

Ecoffey C, Oger E, Marchand-Maillet F, et al. (2014) Complications associated with 27,031 ultrasound-guided axillary brachial plexus blocks. *Eur J Anaesthesiol.* 31,1–5.

Ferraro LH, Takeda A, dos Reis Falcão LF, et al. (2014) Determination of the minimum effective volume of 0.5% bupivacaine for ultrasound-guided axillary brachial plexus block. *Braz J Anesthesiol.* 64,49–53.

Fisher WJ, Bingham RM, Hall R. (1999) Axillary brachial plexus block for perioperative analgesia in 250 children. *Paediatr Anaesth.* 9,435–8.

Hadzic A, Dilberovic F, Shah S, et al. (2004) Combination of intraneural injection and high injection pressure leads to fascicular injury and neurologic deficits in dogs. *Reg Anesth Pain Med.* 29(5),417–23.

Hogan QH. (2008) Pathophysiology of peripheral nerve injury during regional anesthesia. *Reg Anesth Pain Med.* 33,435–41.

Kapur E, Vuckovic I, Dilberovic F, et al. (2007) Neurologic and histologic outcome after intraneural injections of lidocaine in canine sciatic nerves. *Acta Anaesthesiol Scand.* 51,101–7.

McNaught A, Shastri U, Carmichael N, et al. (2011) Ultrasound reduces the minimum effective local anaesthetic volume compared with peripheral nerve stimulation for interscalene block. *Br J Anaesth.* 106,124–30.

Morton, NS, 2004. Local and regional anaesthesia in infants. Continuing education in anaesthesia. *Crit Care Pain.* 4,148–51.

O'Donnell BD, Iohom G. (2009) An estimation of the minimum effective anesthetic volume of 2% lidocaine in ultrasound-guided axillary brachial plexus block. *Anesthesiology.* 111,25–9.

Small GA. (1951) Brachial plexus block anesthesia in children. *JAMA.* 147,1648–51.

Steinfeldt T, Poeschl S, Nimphius W, et al. (2011) Forced needle advancement during needle–nerve contact in a porcine model: histological outcome. *Anesth Analg.*113(2),417–20.

Theroux MC, Dixit D, Brislin R, Como-Fluero S, Sacks S. (2007) Axillary catheter for brachial plexus analgesia in children for postoperative pain control and rigorous physiotherapy – a simple and effective procedure. *Paediatr Anaesth.* 17,302–3.

Thornton KL, Sacks MD, Hall R, Bingham R. (2003) Comparison of 0.2% ropivacaine and 0.25% bupivacaine for axillary brachial plexus blocks in pediatric hand surgery. *Paediatr Anaesth.*13 (5),409–12.

Warren JA, Thoma RB, Georgescu A, Shah SJ. (2007) Intravenous lipid infusion in the successful resuscitation of local anesthetic-induced cardiovascular collapse after supraclavicular brachial plexus block. *Anesth Analg.* 106,1578–80.

Wedel DJ, Krohn JS, Hall JA. (1991) Brachial plexus anaesthesia in pediatric patients. *Mayo Clin Proc.* 66(6),583–8.

Ultrasound-guided supraclavicular brachial plexus block

Mark D. Reisbig

Clinical use

Supraclavicular brachial plexus blockade is becoming more widely utilized in both adult and pediatric patients. A single injection with the supraclavicular approach to brachial plexus blockade can provide complete anesthesia and analgesia for surgical procedures on the upper extremity distal to the shoulder. Supplementation of the block to include the supras-capular nerve branch, which exits the upper trunk (C5–C6) prior to its entry into the supraclavicular fossa, facilitates analgesia for shoulder procedures. Successful blockade of the brachial plexus can reduce opioid consumption and opioid-related side effects, while providing excellent post-operative analgesia. In-depth anatomic knowledge of the brachial plexus and surrounding structures is necessary for efficacious blockade and the prevention of complications.

The supraclavicular blockade of the brachial plexus was first described by the German surgeon, Kulenkampff in 1911 (Kulenkampff, 1911). He found it advantageous that a single injection could anesthetize the entire upper extremity from below the shoulder to the fingers (Kulenkampff and Persky, 1928). Several years later, the first report on a series of brachial plexus blocks on children was published (Small, 1953). In the same time period, a report was made of brachial plexus blocks resulting in serious complications and even death. These complications were attributed to procedural error (Sala De Pablo and Diez-Mallo, 1948). With potentially serious complications in the hands of inexperienced operators, the supraclavicular approach described by Kulenkampff and other "blind" approaches, were never well established in pediatric anesthesiology.

In 1928 Kulenkampff advised, "A *sine qua non* to a proper technique is a clear mental picture of the relation of the structures as they lie under the skin, and a keen sense of direction in which the needle is to be pointed" (Kulenkampff and Persky, 1928). Seventy-five years later, the first ultrasound-guided supraclavicular brachial plexus block technique with needle visualization was described (Chan et al., 2003). Implementation of ultrasound has afforded the anesthesiologist visualization of the needle and local anesthetic (LA) as it traverses the tissues in proximity to the plexus and surrounding structures. Ultrasound-guided techniques have driven increased utilization of the supraclavicular block in pediatric anesthesiology (Polaner et al., 2010). Although the risks of serious complications are still present, ultrasound has added a layer of safety and efficacy to the procedure.

The ultrasound-guided supraclavicular block procedure was first described for pediatric patients aged 5 years and older in 2008 (De Jose Maria et al., 2008). A case series in 2010 later demonstrated safety and efficacy in patients 6 years and younger (Amiri and Espandar, 2010). When compared with the infraclavicular technique, the ultrasound-guided supraclavicular block took less time and is easier to perform in an in-plane fashion due to the position of the clavicle altering the needle path in infraclavicular blockade (Amiri and Espandar, 2010).

In children, supraclavicular blockade can be used for finger, hand, wrist, forearm, elbow, and arm procedures. This block is preferred for many pediatric upper extremity surgeries, as it covers pain caused by the tourniquet and any pain from the surgical procedure itself. An added benefit is post-operative motor blockade, which may reduce risk of damage from movement after delicate hand repairs. Absolute contraindications for supraclavicular blockade are similar to those for all peripheral nerve blocks. These

Ultrasound-Guided Regional Anesthesia in Children, ed. Mannion et al. Published by Cambridge University Press.
© Cambridge University Press 2015.

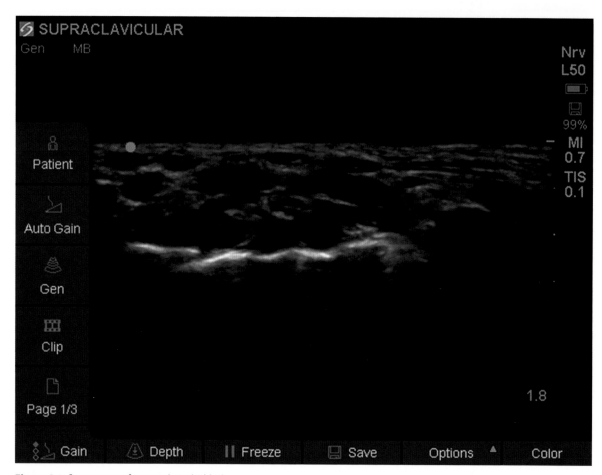

Figure 8.1 Sonoanatomy for supraclavicular block.

include patient or parent refusal, LA allergy, infection at the site of injection, and sepsis. Special consideration should be given to patients with poor respiratory reserve as phrenic nerve paralysis is not uncommon with this block. In addition, the risks and benefits should be considered for patients with contralateral pneumothorax, pneumonectomy, or diaphragmatic paralysis. Other relative contraindications include coagulopathy, neural injury, and contralateral recurrent laryngeal nerve palsy.

Prior to ultrasound guidance for supraclavicular blockade, the risk of pneumothorax and intravascular injection was a major deterrent to performing the block in pediatric cases. Pneumothorax was reported after supraclavicular block at an incidence of 0.5–6.0% in adult populations (Brand and Papper, 1961; Brown et al., 1993). With the advent of ultrasound-guided peripheral nerve blockade, brachial plexus blockade has become most commonly performed at the supraclavicular fossa. Although

limited data exists, no reports of toxicity from intravascular injection or cases of pneumothorax have been reported (Polaner et al., 2010). Other potential untoward effects of supraclavicular blockade that are not uncommon include Horner's syndrome and ipsilateral diaphragmatic paralysis. Although the occurrence of these events is more common in patients receiving interscalene blockade, they should still be considered when deciding to administer a supraclavicular block.

Clinical sonoanatomy

The region to be scanned is just above the clavicle. Inferior to the subclavian artery lies the first rib and the pleura. Superficial to the first rib and lateral to the subclavian artery is where the trunks of the brachial plexus branch to form divisions (Figure 8.1). These appear as a cluster of round hypoechoic masses with hyperechoic rims. The compact anatomic nature of

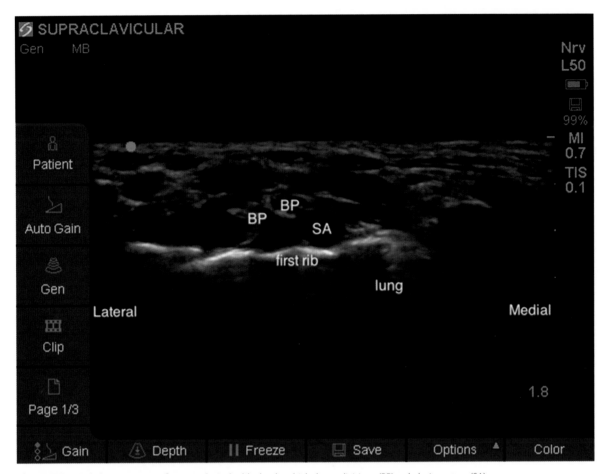

SUPRACLAVICULAR
Gen   MB

Figure 8.2 Labeled sonoanatomy for supraclavicular block – brachial plexus divisions (BP), subclavian artery (SA).

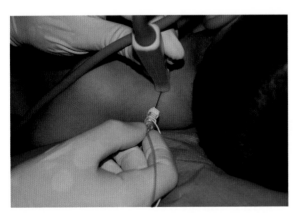

Figure 8.3 Patient position, probe placement, and in-plane needle technique.

the brachial plexus at the supraclavicular fossa allows for a single injection point to reach the nerve to adequately block the arm below the shoulder (Figure 8.2).

Landmarks

The patient should be placed in the supine position with the head turned to the contralateral side. A roll between the scapulae may be necessary in smaller patients. The height of the bed should be set at an ergonomically comfortable level for the anesthesiologist. Placement of the probe is in a coronal-oblique axis along the superior border of the distal clavicle (Figure 8.3). As the probe moves medially, the brachial plexus will come into view lateral to the subclavian artery, above the first rib.

Block performance

A linear, high frequency probe should be placed in the supraclavicular fossa, in the coronal-oblique axis, along the superior border of the distal clavicle. As the probe is guided medially along the clavicle, the hypoechoic subclavian artery should be identified and

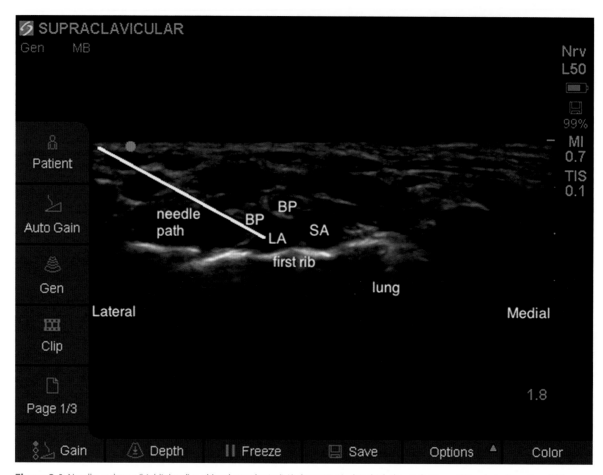

Figure 8.4 Needle pathway (highlighted) and local anesthetic (LA) deposition – brachial plexus divisions (BP), subclavian artery (SA).

the brachial plexus will come into view. Color Doppler should be used to scan for vasculature. With the plexus visualized, the probe should be held in place so that the plexus, first rib, and subclavian artery are all in view. A 22-gauge, 50 mm needle is introduced in-plane from the lateral side to approach the brachial plexus (Figure 8.4). Direct visualization of needle movement is necessary to avoid entering nerve bundles, vasculature, or pleural space. Once in close proximity to the plexus, the syringe should be aspirated as a safety measure to protect against intravascular injection. A small amount of LA should be injected incrementally with re-aspiration of the syringe every 1–2 ml. Redirection of the needle, under direct visualization, with deposition of LA around the entire plexus improves block success and decreases latency. Care should be taken to visualize the needle in-plane at all times, avoiding arterial puncture and placement of the needle below the plexus in the area of the pleura.

A total of 0.25–0.50 ml/kg of 0.25% bupivacaine, 0.25% levobupivacaine, or 0.2% ropivacaine can be used. In patients under 6 months of age, the dose should be reduced by 50%.

Post-operative care

In a patient who has received a supraclavicular block, the extremity must be protected until full function and sensation have returned to the extremity. This includes padding the extremity while lying in bed, or placing the arm in a sling should the patient ambulate. If a child is to be discharged after a day case with residual block, proper education of the parents as well as written instructions are necessary regarding how to care for and protect a weak and numb upper extremity. The parents must also understand how to safely administer oral analgesics prior to the block wearing off to smoothly transition to an oral pain management regimen.

Clinical tips

1. The compact anatomic nature of the brachial plexus at the supraclavicular fossa allows for a single LA injection to block the arm below the shoulder.
2. This block is preferred for many pediatric upper extremity surgeries, as it covers pain caused by the tourniquet.
3. The supraclavicular block should be performed in-plane so as to visualize the needle throughout and so avoid penetration of the vessels or pleura.
4. Common adverse effects of the supraclavicular block include ipsilateral diaphragmatic paralysis and Horner's syndrome.

Suggested reading

Amiri HR, Espandar R. (2010) Upper extremity surgery in younger children under ultrasound-guided supraclavicular brachial plexus block: a case series. *J Child Orthop.* 4,315–19.

Brand L, Papper EM. (1961) A comparison of supraclavicular and axillary techniques for brachial plexus blocks. *Anesthesiology.* 22,226–9.

Brown DL, Cahill DR, Bridenbaugh LD. (1993) Supraclavicular nerve block: anatomic analysis of a method to prevent pneumothorax. *Anesth Analg.* 76,530–4.

Chan VWS, Perlas A, Rawson R, Odukoya O. (2003) Ultrasound-guided supraclavicular brachial plexus block. *Anesth Analg.* 97,1514–17.

De Jose Maria B, Banus E, Egeam MN, et al. (2008) Ultrasound-guided supraclavicular vs. infraclavicular brachial plexus blocks in children. *Paediatr Anaesth.* 18,838–44.

Kulenkampff D. (1911) Anesthesia of the brachial plexus. *Zentralbl Chir.* 38,1337–40.

Kulenkampff D, Persky MA. (1928) Brachial plexus anesthesia: Its indications, technique, and dangers. *Ann Surg.* 87(6),883–91.

Neal JM, Gerancher JC, Hebl JR, et al. (2009) Upper extremity regional anesthesia: Essentials of our current understanding, 2008. *Reg Anesth Pain Med.* 34(2),134–70.

Polaner DM, Taenzer AH, Wakker BJ, et al. (2010) Pediatric regional anesthesia network (PRAN): a multi-institutional study of use and incidence of complications of pediatric regional anesthesia. *Anesth Analg.* 115(6),1353–64.

Sala De Pablo J, Diez-Mallo J. (1948) Experience with three thousand cases of brachial plexus block: its dangers. Report of a fatal case. *Ann Surg.* 128,956–64.

Small GA. (1953) Brachial plexus anesthesia in children. *JAMA.* 147(17),1648–51.

Yang CW, Cho C, Kwon HU, et al. (2010) Ultrasound-guided supraclavicular brachial plexus block in pediatric patients: a report of four cases. *Korean J Anesthesiol.* 59(Suppl),S90–4.

Chapter

9

Ultrasound-guided infraclavicular brachial plexus block

Wallis T. Muhly and Arjunan Ganesh

Clinical use

Several anatomic and nerve stimulator-guided techniques have been reported when approaching the infraclavicular brachial plexus (Raj et al., 1973; Sims, 1977; Borgeat et al., 2001). In recent years ultrasound-guided approaches to the infraclavicular plexus have become increasingly popular (Sandhu and Capan, 2002). Below the clavicle in the infraclavicular fossa, the brachial plexus (BP) is arranged into the lateral, medial, and posterior cords. The musculocutaneous, the axillary, and the medial cutaneous nerves all arise from the plexus in this region. Thus, blockade of the BP within the infraclavicular fossa allows for effective block of all nerves of the upper and lower arm with the exception of the intercostobrachial nerve which arises from T2. As such, the infraclavicular BP block is an appropriate and effective regional technique for surgery on the arm, elbow, forearm, and hand.

Block of the plexus at infraclavicular level has several advantages compared to other techniques, including a lower likelihood of tourniquet pain during surgery, more reliable blockade of the musculocutaneous nerve compared to single injection axillary block, and a significantly shorter block performance time compared to multi-injection axillary or mid-humeral blocks (Chin et al., 2013). Additionally, because of the increased depth at which the plexus is encountered compared to the supraclavicular or axillary approach, placement and securing of a continuous catheter may be easier when using the infraclavicular approach. This may be especially important in children whose increased activity level can increase the possibility of catheter dislodgement.

There is evidence that the use of regional anesthesia for surgery on the upper extremity is not infrequent in children. The recently published prospective, observational multicenter study of regional anesthesia

practice patterns in the United States published by the Pediatric Regional Anesthesia Network (PRAN) revealed that, of the 14 917 blocks performed over a 3-year period, 3% of blocks were performed for upper extremity surgery (Polaner et al., 2012). Of the 455 single-injection blocks performed on the upper extremity, the infraclavicular approach accounted for 40 blocks and of the 26 upper extremity continuous catheters reported, 8 were performed at the infraclavicular position. In 2010, the survey of the French-Language Society of Pediatric Anesthesiologists (ADARPEF) reported on 31 132 regional anesthetics performed in children (Ecoffey et al., 2010). Upper extremity blocks accounted for 6.7% of all blocks, and the infraclavicular approach accounted for 11% of upper extremity blocks or 0.8% of all blocks.

Only a handful of case reports or case series have been reported on the use of infraclavicular BP blocks in children (Dadure et al., 2003, Fleischmann et al., 2003; Fisher et al., 2006). These reports consistently demonstrate that the infraclavicular space is a suitable approach for both single injection and continuous perineural infusions. In addition to routine post-operative analgesia indications, there are case reports of the value of infraclavicular continuous perineural catheters in the setting of pediatric limb salvage surgery and neonatal limb ischemia (Loland et al., 2009; Ponde et al., 2012). While the indications for use of this technique are not as clear as in the adult setting, it is a useful technique in the appropriate clinical setting. We will review the specifics of block performance in the following sections.

Clinical sonoanatomy

The infraclavicular BP runs within the infraclavicular fossa which is bordered anteriorly by the pectoralis major and minor muscles, superiorly by the clavicle and coracoid process, medially by the ribs and laterally

Ultrasound-Guided Regional Anesthesia in Children, ed. Mannion et al. Published by Cambridge University Press.
© Cambridge University Press 2015.

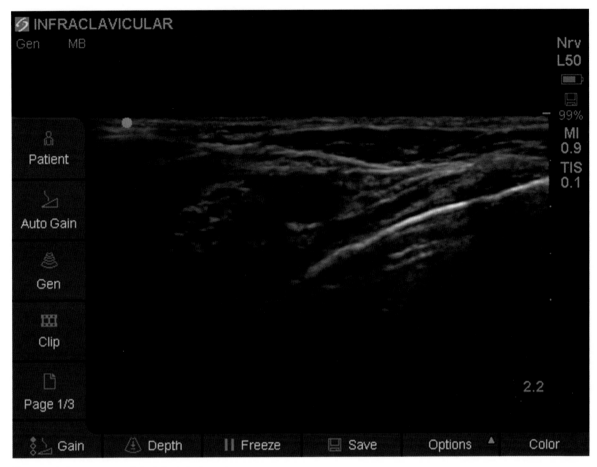

Figure 9.1 Sonoanatomy of the infraclavicular region.

by the humerus (Figure 9.1). As stated above the BP is arranged into the lateral, medial, and posterior cords, so named for their position relative to the axillary artery (Figure 9.2). The musculocutaneous nerve arises from the lateral cord at the level of the pectoralis minor muscle, the axillary nerve from the posterior cord at the level of the coracoid and the medial cutaneous nerve from the medial cord.

The key anatomic structure to identify is the axillary artery lying posterior to the pectoralis major and minor muscles (Figure 9.2). Although a great deal of anatomic variability exists, the lateral cord is typically located superior to the artery while the posterior and medial cords are located posterior and inferior to the artery respectively.

Landmarks

The patient should be placed in the supine position. The transducer is placed in a parasagittal position below the clavicle on the medial aspect of the coracoid process

(Figure 9.3). Depending on the size and body habitus of the child, a probe with a short linear length such as 25 mm may be required. Some adjustment of the probe in multiple planes may be necessary to achieve a satisfactory view of the artery and the surrounding cords. Abduction of the arm to 90 degrees may be helpful by moving the acromioclavicular junction superiorly.

Block performance

In younger or thin children a high frequency linear probe may be sufficient for visualization of the infraclavicular fossa while a lower frequency curved array probe may be necessary in larger children and adolescents to visualize a deeper infraclavicular fossa. Color Doppler may be useful to verify the position of the axillary artery and vein.

The lateral cord is seen as a hyperechoic structure as is the posterior cord, which can be seen posterior to the axillary artery at the 6 o'clock position. The medial cord may be more difficult to visualize but the

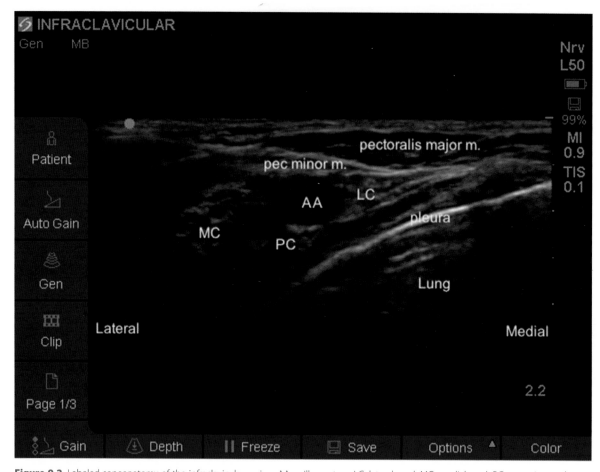

Figure 9.2 Labeled sonoanatomy of the infraclavicular region. AA, axillary artery; LC, lateral cord; MC, medial cord; PC, posterior cord.

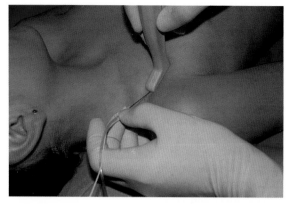

Figure 9.3 Probe position, which may need to be adjusted to obtain the best view that still permits a lateral to medial needle approach. Abduction of the arm may help by moving the coracoid process superiorly and laterally.

injection of 1–2 ml of LA anterior to the artery may improve its localization.

For single injection a 22-gauge needle can be used and the length of needle (50–100 mm) can be chosen based on the child's size and plexus depth. A 25 mm BP needle may be sufficient in infants and small children while a 100 mm BP needle may be required to reach the infraclavicular fossa in adolescents.

The needle is then inserted between the coracoid process and the superior portion of the ultrasound probe. The needle is advanced in-plane through the pectoralis major and minor muscles (Figure 9.4). Because of the steep needle angle required to reach the infraclavicular BP, the needle image may not be very clear so care must be taken to monitor tissue displacement as the needle is advanced in an effort to avoid puncturing the artery. The LA is injected in small 3–5 ml increments around the cords ensuring that there is adequate perivascular spread of the LA,

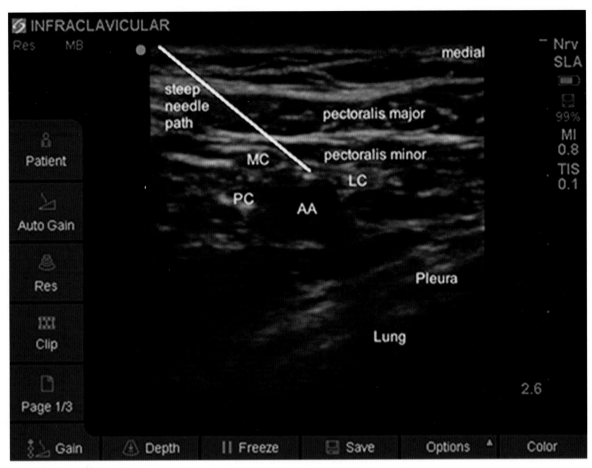

Figure 9.4 Needle path highlighted. In practice the steep angle required may make needle visualization difficult. AA, axillary artery; LC, lateral cord; MC, medial cord; PC, posterior cord.

especially medially and laterally around the artery. Current recommended volumes are 0.5 ml/kg of 0.2% ropivacaine or 0.25% bupivacaine, although these volumes may reduce with the increasing experience with ultrasound to guide LA deposition for this block.

If placing a catheter, the use of a short 50 mm Touhy needle in infants and younger children and a 100 mm Touhy needle in young adults would be appropriate. Ideally, the catheter should be placed at the 6 o'clock position adjacent to the posterior cord where the infusate can reach both the medial and lateral cords. Several methods have been described to verify catheter position including the injection of agitated 5% dextrose (Dhir and Ganapathy, 2008) or the injection of a small amount of air (Kan et al., 2013). Once the catheter is in position, LA is injected with ultrasound visualization in 3–5 ml increments following careful aspiration of the catheter. In order

to ensure complete BP coverage, medial and lateral extension of the local anesthetic around the axillary artery should be present. The catheter is then carefully secured to the patient. A single drop of dermabond applied to the catheter insertion site helps reduce the possibility of catheter dislodgement and/or pericatheter leakage (Gurnaney et al., 2011). The catheter can then be affixed to the patient using a sterile non-occlusive dressing.

For continuous peripheral nerve blockade an infusion of ropivacaine (0.4 mg/kg/h) or bupivacaine (0.4 mg/kg/h) is commenced with a typical maximum infusion rate of 8–10 ml/h.

Post-operative care

Children and adolescents can be safely discharged home following regional anesthesia (Gurnaney et al.,

2014). In the case of single shot peripheral nerve block, it is important to prepare the patient's parents for the eventual resolution of the block and the potential for increased pain and anxiety in the child. This can be quite alarming to families if not adequately prepared, and a plan for oral analgesics should be available and reviewed with the family prior to discharge. Additionally, it is appropriate to follow up the patient who had a single shot nerve block the following day to confirm resolution of the sensory block and also to monitor for any complications. When a continuous perineural catheter is placed, we recommend daily follow-up phone calls or hospital visits for inpatients to monitor patient response until the catheter has been removed and the block has resolved (Gurnaney et al., 2014). This type of support can relieve parental concerns about managing LA infusions at home and provide a resource for families as they recover from their surgical procedure.

> **Clinical tips**
> - Ultrasound-guided infraclavicular block allows for complete brachial plexus blockade.
> - The axillary artery is the key sonographic landmark.
> - This block is ideally suited for placement of a catheter for continuous post-operative analgesia.
> - The injection of small volumes of LA can improve the localization of the three cords.
> - Ensuring sufficient perivascular spread of LA will significantly increase the success rate of the block

Suggested reading

Borgeat A, Ekatodramis G, Dumont C. (2001) An evaluation of the infraclavicular block via a modified approach of the Raj technique. *Anesth Analg.* 93,436–41.

Chin, KJ, Alakkad H, Adhikary SD, Singh M. (2013) Infraclavicular brachial plexus block for regional anaesthesia of the lower arm. *Cochrane Database Syst Rev.* 8, CD005487.

Dadure C, Raux O, Troncin R, Rochette A, Capdevila X. (2003) Continuous infraclavicular brachial plexus block for acute pain management in children. *Anesth Analg.* 97,691–3.

Dhir S, Ganapathy S. (2008) Use of ultrasound guidance and contrast enhancement: a study of continuous infraclavicular brachial plexus approach. *Acta Anaesthesiol Scand.* 52,338–42.

Ecoffey C, Lacroix F, Giaufre E, Orliaguet G, Courreges P; Association des anesthesistes reanimateurs pediatriques d'expression Française. (2010) Epidemiology and morbidity of regional anesthesia in children: a follow-up one-year prospective survey of the French-Language Society of Paediatric Anaesthesiologists (ADARPEF). *Paediatr Anaesth.* 20,1061–9.

Fisher P, Wilson SE, Brown M, Ditunno T. (2006) Continuous infraclavicular brachial plexus block in a child. *Paediatr Anaesth.* 16,884–6.

Fleischmann E, Marhofer P, Greher M, et al. (2003) Brachial plexus anaesthesia in children: lateral infraclavicular vs. axillary approach. *Paediatr Anaesth.* 13,103–8.

Gurnaney H, Kraemer FW, Ganesh A. (2011) Dermabond decreases pericatheter local anesthetic leakage after continuous perineural infusions. *Anesth Analg.* 113,206.

Gurnaney H, Kraemer FW, Maxwell L, et al. (2014) Ambulatory continuous peripheral nerve blocks in children and adolescents: a longitudinal 8-year single center study. *Anesth Analg.* 118,621–7.

Kan JM, Harrison TK, Kim TE, et al. (2013) An in vitro study to evaluate the utility of the "air test" to infer perineural catheter tip location. *J Ultrasound Med.* 32,529–33.

Loland VJ, Ilfeld BM, Abrams RA, Mariano ER. (2009) Ultrasound-guided perineural catheter and local anesthetic infusion in the perioperative management of pediatric limb salvage: a case report. *Paediatr Anaesth.* 19,905–7.

Polaner DM, Taenzer AH, Walker BJ, et al. (2012) Pediatric Regional Anesthesia Network (PRAN): a multi-institutional study of the use and incidence of complications of pediatric regional anesthesia. *Anesth Analg.* 115,1353–64.

Ponde VC, Shah DM, Mane S. (2012) Role of ultrasound-guided continuous brachial plexus block in the management of neonatal ischemia in upper limb. *Saudi J Anaesth.* 6,423–5.

Raj PP, Montgomery SJ, Nettles D, Jenkins MT. (1973) Infraclavicular brachial plexus block-a new approach. *Anesth Analg.* 52,897–904.

Sandhu NS, Capan LM. (2002) Ultrasound-guided infraclavicular brachial plexus block. *Br J Anaesth.* 89,254–9.

Sims JK. (1977) A modification of landmarks for infraclavicular approach to brachial plexus block. *Anesth Analg.* 56,554–5.

Chapter

10

Ultrasound-guided interscalene brachial plexus block

Harshad Gurnaney and Arjunan Ganesh

Clinical use

Regional anesthesia of the upper extremity can be achieved by placing local anesthetic (LA) at varying locations along the course of the brachial plexus. The brachial plexus begins just outside the intervertebral foramina at the lower cervical region from the ventral rami of C5–C8 and T1 spinal nerves. The C5 and C6 rami join to form the superior trunk at the lateral border of the middle scalene muscle; the C8 and T1 rami join to form the inferior trunk, and the C7 ramus continues as the middle trunk. These trunks lie between the anterior and middle scalene muscles and neural blockade at this site is termed the interscalene brachial plexus or interscalene block (ISB).

ISB has demonstrated efficacy in providing post-operative analgesia after shoulder and proximal humerus surgery. The use of ISB is associated with a reduction in post-operative pain scores, opioid requirements, and opioid-related side effects after shoulder surgery.

It is generally considered to be superior to the supraclavicular block for shoulder procedures as it provides coverage of the suprascapular nerve, which provides sensation to the shoulder joint.

The common complications of the ISB are Horner's syndrome (block of the cervical sympathetic chain leading to ptosis, miosis and anhidrosis on the ipsilateral side) and phrenic nerve block which can lead to shortness of breath. A rare but potentially devastating complication of the ISB is injury to the cervical spinal cord. The American Society of Regional Anesthesia (ASRA), in its guidelines for performing regional anesthesia for patients under general anesthesia, recommended that the ISB not be placed while a patient is under general anesthesia (Bernards et al., 2008). One of the reasons for this recommendation is the risk of spinal cord damage during an ISB secondary to the needle entry into the spinal canal (Benumof, 2000). A majority of the peripheral nerve blocks in pediatric patients are placed with the patient under general anesthesia (Gurnaney et al., 2014). In addition, placement of an ISB with a pediatric patient awake or under mild sedation carries the risk of patient movement during the procedure while the needle is in close proximity to important neurovascular structures in the neck. A recent study of 518 ISBs in children with 390 performed under general anesthetic and 123 performed with the patient sedated or awake, found no postoperative neurologic symptoms or complications (Taenzer et al., 2014).

In two recent reports ultrasound guidance was found to be superior to nerve stimulation in placing the ISB and continuous interscalene catheter (Kapral et al., 2008; Fredrickson et al., 2009). Kapral et al. reported that surgical anesthesia was achieved in 99% of patients in the ultrasound group compared to 91% in the nerve stimulation group. Fredrickson et al. reported reduction in proportion of patients requiring opioids and reduction in catheter interventions (patient-administered boluses) on postoperative day 1 for catheters placed using ultrasound guidance. These differences did not continue into post-operative day 2. The use of ultrasound guidance could help in identifying anatomic variations in the position of the roots of the brachial plexus; for example, in a small percentage of patients the nerve roots lie within the belly of the anterior scalene muscle (Natsis et al., 2006). Ultrasound guidance provides a mean for visualizing the spread of LA around the target nerves and provides confirmation of the needle tip location throughout the injection of LA, whereas the nerve simulation only provides initial confirmation of the needle tip location in the proximity of the nerve and is abolished once 1–2 ml of LA is injected.

Ultrasound-Guided Regional Anesthesia in Children, ed. Mannion et al. Published by Cambridge University Press.
© Cambridge University Press 2015.

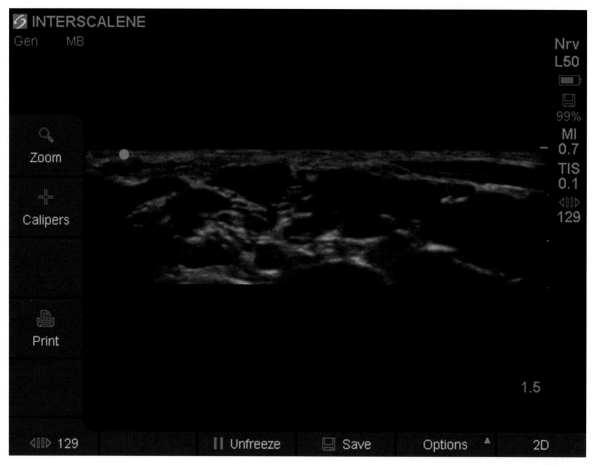

Figure 10.1 Sonoanatomy for interscalene block (ISB).

Clinical sonoanatomy

The C5–C7 nerve roots are located at approximately the level of the sixth/seventh cervical vertebrae in the interscalene groove, which is formed by the anterior and middle scalene muscles (Figure 10.1). The nerve roots are close to the lateral edge of the sternocleidomastoid muscle and the external jugular vein. While performing this block care should be taken to avoid needle entry into the external jugular vein.

Landmarks

The patient is positioned supine with the head slightly rotated to the contralateral side on a pillow (Figure 10.2). The cricoid cartilage can be used as a landmark to identify the C5/6 vertebral level.

Block performance

A high frequency probe should be used with the depth set to 2–3 cm, as the nerve roots are located superficially. The probe is placed about 2 cm cephalad and parallel to the clavicle. A slight caudal or cephalad tilting of the ultrasound probe may help improve visualization of the brachial plexus in the interscalene groove. A 25 mm needle is recommended for most children as the plexus is very superficial. A tangential caudal oriented needle approach from lateral to medial direction to the plexus is recommended to reduce the risk of needle injury to the spinal cord (Figure 10.2). The needle can be inserted in-plane or out-of-plane. The in-plane approach is described here. Firstly, the anterior and middle scalene muscles and the cervical nerve roots are visualized in the short axis (Figure 10.3). The needle is then advanced in a lateral to medial direction until the needle tip is located in the interscalene groove just lateral to the superficial brachial plexus nerve roots (Figure 10.4).

Once the needle tip is in the correct position up to 0.5 ml/kg of 0.2% ropivacaine is injected under ultrasound guidance (maximum of 20 ml).

Continuous catheter technique

The modified lateral approach is the common technique for placement of a continuous ISB catheter (Borgeat et al., 2003). The patient position and probe orientation are similar to that of a single injection technique. Once the needle is positioned in the interscalene groove the needle tip location can be confirmed with nerve stimulation or by injecting a small amount of dextrose 5% through the needle (Fredrickson et al., 2009). This will help confirm that the needle tip is in the interscalene groove and also ease the advancement of the catheter into the interscalene space. The next part of the procedure is to maintain the needle position while inserting a

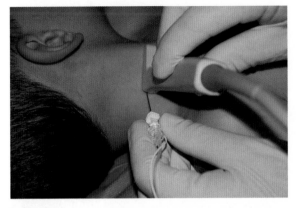

Figure 10.2 Patient position, probe placement, and in-plane needle approach.

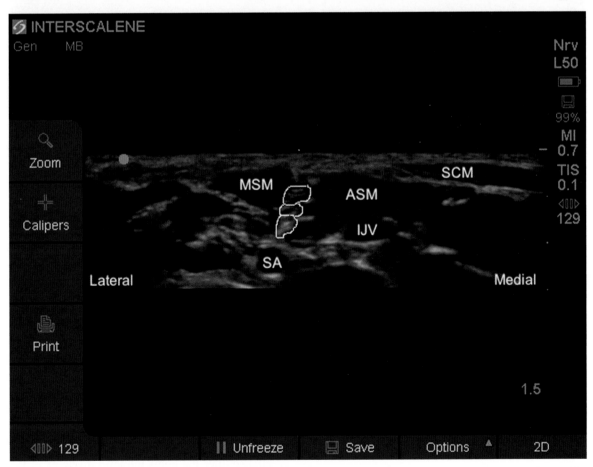

Figure 10.3 Labeled sonoanatomy for interscalene block (ISB). The roots of the brachial plexus are outlined. ASM, anterior scalene muscle; IJV, internal jugular vein; MSM, middle scalene muscle; SA, subclavian artery; SCM, sternocleidomastoid muscle.

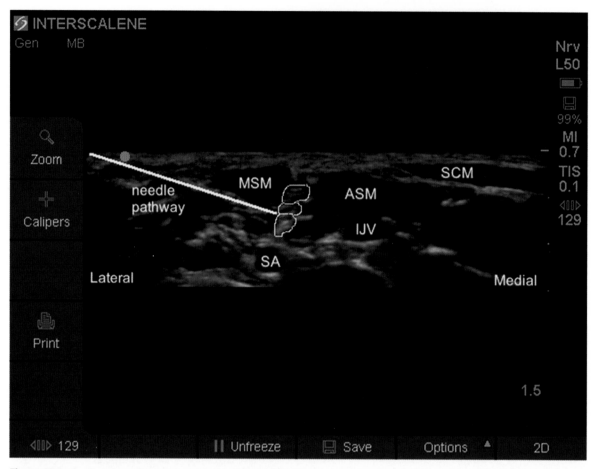

Figure 10.4 Needle pathway for in-plane interscalene block (ISB). ASM, anterior scalene muscle; IJV, internal jugular vein; MSM, middle scalene muscle; SA, subclavian artery; SCM, sternocleidomastoid muscle.

catheter through the needle. If continuous ultrasound visualization is sought a second operator is needed to help pass the catheter. Once the catheter is inserted the catheter tip position is confirmed by visualizing an injection of a small amount of LA through the catheter. Following this confirmation the intended dose of LA is administered through the catheter. As these catheters are relatively superficial it is important to secure the catheter well to avoid accidental dislodgement. Catheters may be tunneled to decrease the risk of dislodgement. A drop of dermabond at the catheter insertion site can help reduce pericatheter leakage and help secure the catheter (Gurnaney et al., 2011). The catheter is secured using an adhesive skin preparation followed by a clear dressing to allow inspection of the catheter insertion site.

Post-operative care

The parents and child should be warned preoperatively about the potential for Horner's syndrome with this block. In addition the risk of ipsilateral phrenic nerve block can lead to ventilatory compromise in children with a history of moderate to severe lung disease. A single injection block is expected to last 12–18 hours, and an analgesia plan should be in place for when the block resolves. The parents and child should be warned about the risk of temporary paresthesias and dysesthesias after an ISB as the risk is higher for the ISB (2–3%) compared to other brachial plexus blocks.

Continuous infusion for an interscalene catheter is initiated after the bolus intraoperatively or in the recovery room. Dilute bupivacaine, levobupivacaine or ropivacaine are used for the infusion. An infusion rate of 0.10–0.15 ml/kg with a maximum rate of 10 ml/h is recommended for the continuous infusion. Addition of adjuvants has not been beneficial for continuous nerve blocks.

Clinical tips

- The brachial plexus can be identified in the supraclavicular location lateral to the subclavian artery. If the ultrasound probe is moved in a cephalad direction from this location the brachial plexus can be visualized in the interscalene groove.
- The extremely close proximity of vital structures such as the carotid artery, cervical epidural space, and jugular veins must be appreciated.
- Nerve stimulation may be used to confirm the placement of the needle close to the nerves, especially in situations where an optimal image cannot be obtained with the ultrasound.
- Presence of high injection pressure during LA injection may indicate needle to nerve contact and should prompt a slight withdrawal of the needle to avoid injection into the nerve roots.

Suggested reading

Benumof JL. (2000) Permanent loss of cervical spinal cord function associated with interscalene block performed under general anesthesia. *Anesthesiology.* 93,1541–4.

Bernards CM, Hadzic A, Suresh S, Neal JM. (2008) Regional anesthesia in anesthetized or heavily sedated patients. *Reg Anesth Pain Med.* 33,449–60.

Borgeat A, Dullenkopf A, Ekatodramis G, Nagy L. (2003) Evaluation of the lateral modified approach for continuous interscalene block after shoulder surgery. *Anesthesiology.* 99,436–42.

Fredrickson MJ, Ball CM, Dalgleish AJ, Stewart AW, Short TG. (2009) A prospective randomized comparison of ultrasound and neurostimulation as needle end points for interscalene catheter placement. *Anesth Analg.* 108,1695–700.

Gadsden JC, Choi JJ, Lin E, Robinson A. (2014) Opening injection pressure consistently detects needle-nerve contact during ultrasound-guided interscalene brachial plexus block. *Anesthesiology.* 120,1246–53.

Gurnaney H, Kraemer FW, Ganesh A. (2011) Dermabond decreases pericatheter local anesthetic leakage after continuous perineural infusions. *Anesth Analg.* 113,206.

Gurnaney H, Kraemer FW, Maxwell L, et al. (2014) Ambulatory continuous peripheral nerve blocks in children and adolescents: a longitudinal 8-year single center study. *Anesth Analg.* 118,621–7.

Kapral S, Greher M, Huber G, et al. (2008) Ultrasonographic guidance improves the success rate of interscalene brachial plexus blockade. *Reg Anesth Pain Med.* 33,253–8.

Natsis K, Totlis T, Tsikaras P, et al. (2006) Variations of the course of the upper trunk of the brachial plexus and their clinical significance for the thoracic outlet syndrome: a study on 93 cadavers. *Am Surg.* 72,188–92.

Taenzer A, Walker BJ, Bosenberg AT, et al. (2014) Interscalene brachial plexus blocks under general anesthesia in children: is this safe practice? A report from the Pediatric Regional Anesthesia Network (PRAN). *Reg Anesth Pain Med.* 39, 502–5.

Chapter 11

Ultrasound-guided femoral nerve block

Frédéric Duflo

Clinical use

Femoral nerve block (FNB) under ultrasound guidance is very popular among pediatric anesthesiologists or emergency department physicians to efficaciously relieve pain after femoral shaft fracture or hip and knee surgery (Dadure et al., 2009; Flack and Anderson, 2012; Frenkel et al., 2012).

Once the FNB is performed the quadriceps muscle, periosteum and the skin of front of thigh and the medial aspect of the knee, leg, ankle and foot are usually anesthetized.

Compared with neurostimulation, ultrasound-guided FNB results in greater success rates, permits a 50% reduction in local anesthetic (LA) volume and displays prolonged analgesia (Oberndorfer et al., 2007; Ponde et al., 2013). In addition, ultrasound-guided FNB can be performed when neurostimulation is hampered by certain circumstances, i.e. concurrent use of neuromuscular-blocking drugs, arthrogryposis, joint immobilization, muscles disorders, or fractured lower limb when eliciting painful muscle movements should be avoided (Oberndorfer et al., 2007; Dadure et al., 2009). Another advantage of an ultrasound approach is to clearly visualize and identify the vessels or soft tissue of primary importance (Flack and Anderson, 2012).

Clinical sonoanatomy

The femoral nerve is formed from anterior branches of the L2, L3, and L4 spinal nerves before exiting the pelvis and entering the thigh under the inguinal ligament (Figure 11.1). The femoral artery and vein lie immediately medially to the nerve in the configuration nerve, artery, vein, or NAV. The femoral nerve appears triangle or sail-like and is superficial to the quadriceps muscles (Figure 11.2).

Landmarks

Depending on whether the anesthesiologist is right- or left-handed, the ultrasound machine is generally placed to the opposite side of the operator and the practitioner faces the screen. With the child usually in the supine position, the femoral region is best visualized when the lower limb is slightly abducted with external rotation. Under ultrasound guidance, a high-frequency linear array probe is positioned in the inguinal crease (parallel and just below the inguinal ligament) and placed perpendicular to the nerve axis (Figure 11.3). After a transverse back and forth scan (with gentle slide/tilt/rotation), the femoral nerve is easily located laterally to the femoral artery (the latter appearing as an anechoic circular non-compressive pulsatile structure; Doppler ultrasound might be helpful to identify the femoral artery for beginners). Ultrasound guidance may reduce the risk of femoral artery puncture compared with conventional techniques. The profunda femoris artery or the superficial iliac circumflex artery might be visualized if the probe is cranially or caudally applied to the femoral region. The femoral nerve appears as a rough triangle-shaped hyperechoic structure lying on the iliopsoas muscle sulcus at a 1–2 cm depth and covered by the fascia iliaca. With a certain expertise, the practitioner can locate the femoral nerve lying below both fascias lata and iliaca separately, encountered at this level as thin hyperechoic layers, and the easily collapsed femoral vein. (A gentle pressure exerted by the operator of the probe on the patent is highly recommended to prevent femoral vein collapse and may improve visualization.)

The femoral nerve is usually greatly sensitive to anisotropy (i.e. change in ultrasound direction), and one must frequently adjust cranially and caudally the transducer to optimize correct visualization of the

Ultrasound-Guided Regional Anesthesia in Children, ed. Mannion et al. Published by Cambridge University Press.
© Cambridge University Press 2015.

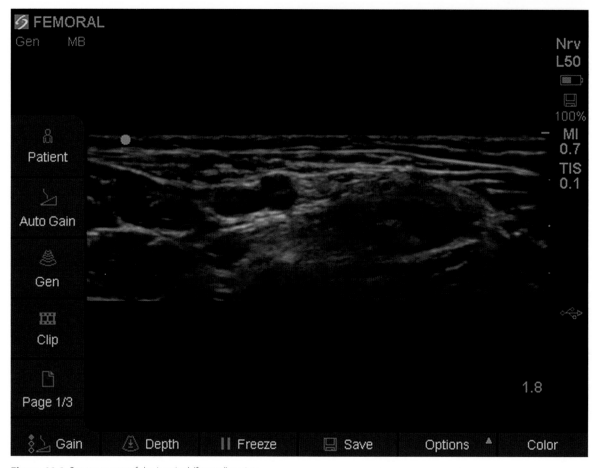

Figure 11.1 Sonoanatomy of the inguinal (femoral) region.

femoral region and accurately distinguish musculo-skeletal and nerve structures. For coverage of the medial/lateral aspects of the lower limb and depending on surgical incision location, the practitioner should consider combining the FNB with either a lateral femoral cutaneous nerve block, sciatic nerve block, or obturator nerve block.

Block performance

Depending on body weight or anatomy of the child, a 25, 50, or 100-mm 22-gauge echoic needle is generally used, and a transducer probe with a small footprint habitually facilitates block performance in infants or toddlers.

After sterile preparation of the site, and most commonly under general anesthesia or local infiltration, the block needle is inserted and advanced under ultrasound guidance. After optimizing the femoral nerve view, the shaft needle is usually best visualized in the long axis (Figure 11.4).

The needle tip is advanced in an "in-plane" manner towards the lateral side of the femoral nerve after penetrating both fascias and the LA is customarily deposited below and laterally to the femoral nerve after test aspiration. Studies evaluating LA spread are lacking in the pediatric population, i.e. above/below or circumferential of LA diffusion. The LA should be injected once the first layer of the fascia iliaca is penetrated, above the femoral branches division and adjacent to the posterolateral or anterior aspects of the femoral nerve. The deposited LA solution spreads as a hypoechoic collection while sheath distention is observed and femoral nerve echogenicity is increased. Some practitioners systematically scan the femoral region proximally and distally to assess the extent of the injectate. The injection of the solution must be executed without resistance; in that case, repositioning the needle tip is mandatory to prevent intrafascicular injection. The LA usually spreads superficially above

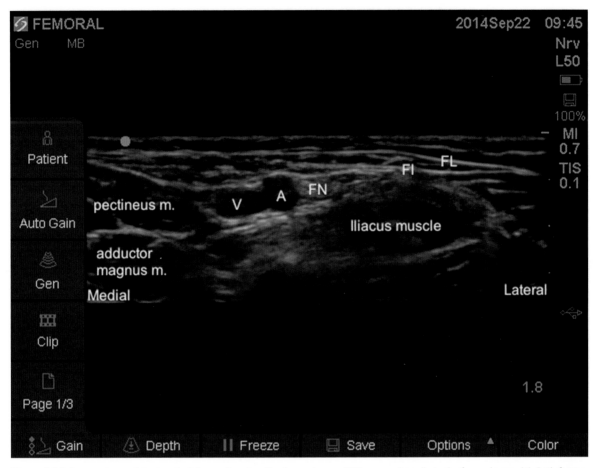

Figure 11.2 Sonoanatomy of the inguinal (femoral) region. The femoral nerve (FN) appears laterally to the femoral artery (A). Both fasciae (lata – FL and iliaca – FI) can be visualized. The femoral vein (V) is commonly visualized medially to both the femoral artery and nerve.

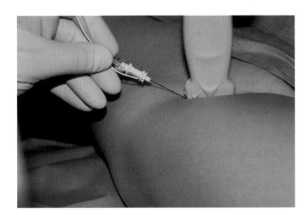

Figure 11.3 Probe placement and patient position.

the femoral nerve unless the needle tip is located in the wedge-shaped fascia iliaca.

The optimal volume of LA has not been evaluated for this block in children, but a volume of 0.2 ml/kg is recommended.

An out-of-plane technique has been described but has mostly not favored pediatric anesthesiologists, because tracking the needle tip can be challenging in that situation.

A South African study supports an ultrasound approach in comparison with nerve stimulator guidance in a study of 14 children (Oberndorfer et al., 2007). The use of ultrasound was associated with increased success rate and prolonged duration of sensory blockade with reduced amounts of LA (0.15 vs. 0.30 ml/kg of levobupivacaine 0.5%). In adults though, using that approach, more nerve needle contact might occur with potential adverse neurologic nerve events (Ruiz et al., 2014).

Finally, depending on surgical incision location, deliberate injection of additional volume may lead to lateral spread underneath the fascia iliaca and block-ade of the lateral femoral cutaneous nerve (Flack et al., 2012). Miller has recently described a combined

87

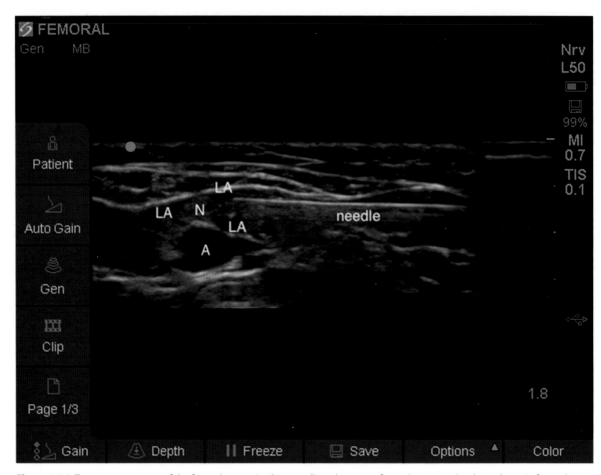

Figure 11.4 Transverse sonogram of the femoral region. In-plane needle technique. A, femoral artery; LA, local anesthetic; N, femoral nerve.

femoral nerve and lateral femoral cutaneous nerve blockade under ultrasound guidance using the same needle (Miller, 2011a). In brief, once the femoral nerve is blocked, the transducer is moved laterally along the inguinal ligament and the lateral femoral cutaneous nerve is identified between both fascia lata and iliaca layers above the sartorius muscle; 1–2 ml of LA solution is suffice to surround nerve branches.

Ultrasound-guided fascia iliaca block

In children, the femoral nerve can also be blocked using the ultrasound-guided fascia iliaca compartment block approach. An in-plane long-axis approach directed cephalad has been recently described for the first time by Miller in three children undergoing hip or femur surgery and appears a reliable and successful procedure for pain relief (Miller, 2011b). The needle tip was placed just below the fascia iliaca into the iliacus muscle. However, as a case report study, there has been no evaluation

of the minimum volume of LA required. Rather, a 0.63–0.80 ml/kg ropivacaine 0.2% single shot has been injected in these cases. Further studies are required to clearly demonstrate efficacy in this promising technique.

Femoral nerve blockade

Placement of a femoral nerve catheter for continuous infusion under ultrasound guidance is carried out in the same manner and offers efficacious pain relief. In- or out-of-plane short-axis approach insertion is at the discretion of the practitioner and no study has compared both techniques.

Post-operative care

In a patient who has received a FNB, the extremity must be protected until full function and sensation have returned to the extremity. This may include bed rest; mobilization should only occur with the support and assistance of at least one other person until such time as normal sensation, proprioception, and motor function return. The resulting quadriceps weakness can contribute to falls. If a child is to be discharged as a day case with residual block, proper education of the parents as well as written instructions are necessary regarding how to care for and protect a weak and numb lower extremity. The parents must also understand how to safely administer oral analgesics prior to the block wearing off to smoothly transition to an oral pain management regimen.

> **Clinical tips**
> * Patients should mobilize with another person until full block resolution to avoid the risk of falls.
> * The femoral nerve block can be combined with a sciatic or popliteal block to provide complete lower leg anesthesia and analgesia.
> * The femoral nerve block is ideal for catheter placement and continuous regional anesthesia.
> * Obturator nerve blockade does not occur as part of a femoral nerve block in most cases.

Suggested reading

Dadure C, Raux O, Rochette A, Capdevila X. (2009) Interest of ultrasonographic guidance in pediatric regional anaesthesia. *Ann Fr Anesth Reanim.* 28,878–84.

Flack S, Anderson C. (2012) Ultrasound guided lower extremity blocks. *Paediatr Anaesth.* 22, 72–80.

Frenkel O, Mansour K, Fisher JW. (2012) Ultrasound-guided femoral nerve block for pain control in an infant with a femur fracture due to nonaccidental trauma. *Pediatr Emerg Care.* 28,183–4.

Miller BR. (2011a) Combined ultrasound-guided femoral and lateral femoral cutaneous nerve blocks in pediatric patients requiring surgical repair of femur fractures. *Paediatr Anaesth.* 21,1163–4.

Miller BR. (2011b) Ultrasound-guided fascia iliaca compartment block in pediatric patients using a long-axis, in-plane needle technique: a report of three cases. *Paediatr Anaesth.* 21,1261–4.

Oberndorfer U, Marhofer P, Bösenberg A, et al.(2007)Ultrasonographic guidance for sciatic and femoral nerve blocks in children. *Br J Anaesth.* 98,797–801.

Ponde V, Desai AP, Shah D. (2013) Comparison of success rate of ultrasound-guided sciatic and femoral nerve block and neurostimulation in children with arthrogryposis multiplex congenita: a randomized clinical trial. *Paediatr Anaesth.* 23,74–8.

Ruiz A, Sal-Blanch X, Martinez-Ocón J, et al. (2014) Incidence of intraneural needle insertion in ultrasound-guided femoral nerve block: a comparison between the out-of-plane versus the in-plane approaches. *REDAR* 61,73–7.

Tsui B, Suresh S. (2010) Ultrasound imaging for regional anesthesia in infants, children, and adolescents: a review of current literature and its application in the practice of extremity and trunk blocks. *Anesthesiology.* 112,473–92.

Chapter

12

Ultrasound-guided saphenous nerve block

Ahmed Abdel-Aziz and Amr Abdelaal

Clinical use

Saphenous nerve blockade is useful for analgesia after knee surgery as part of a multimodal approach (Flack and Anderson, 2012). The saphenous nerve is mainly a sensory nerve (Hebl and Lennon, 2010). The saphenous nerve block, unlike the femoral nerve block, has significantly less motor blockade of the quadriceps as only the vastus medialis is affected, thus allowing early mobilization and rehabilitation (Kim et al., 2014).

It is useful for operations on the anteromedial and posteromedial aspect of the leg from the knee to the ankle (Kent et al., 2013). It may be performed in combination with a popliteal block for ankle surgery.

The saphenous nerve block is increasingly replacing the femoral nerve block for analgesia after knee surgery including total arthroplasty (Kim et al., 2014).

The use of ultrasound guidance for saphenous nerve block is relatively new (Krombach and Gray, 2007) with limited experience in pediatric practice.

The commonest clinical use in children is for knee arthroscopic diagnostic and treatment surgeries.

The anatomy of the saphenous nerve is such that it is accessible for ultrasound-guided blocks at multiple points in the thigh (Hunter et al., 1979; Kent et al., 2013).

Clinical sonoanatomy

The saphenous nerve is the largest cutaneous branch of the femoral nerve and is considered its terminal branch from the posterior division of the femoral nerve. It travels with the femoral artery down the medial aspect of the leg giving off an infrapatellar branch that provides innervation to the skin covering the knee. The saphenous nerve then exits between the sartorius muscle and gracilis tendon and continues down to supply the anteromedial aspect of the leg usually until the medial malleolus (although its sensory innervation may extend beyond the malleolus to the medial aspect of the foot).

The ultrasound image will depend on where along the inner thigh the probe is placed and, therefore, the relationship of the nerve with the femoral artery (Figure 12.1). In the proximal third of the thigh the saphenous nerve separates from the femoral artery after crossing it from lateral to medial. It then courses through the adductor canal (also called subsartorial canal or Hunter canal) with the femoral artery, and emerges from the canal with the saphenous branch of the descending genicular artery.

The canal is bounded anteriorly by the sartorius muscle, antero-laterally by the vastus medialis and postero-medially by the adductor muscles (Figure 12.2). The canal contains the femoral artery and vein, the descending genicular and muscular branches of the femoral artery, the saphenous nerve, and the nerve to vastus medialis.

The saphenous nerve can be identified adjacent to the artery. It may be difficult to visualize as it is very small. It is usually hyperechoic and typically creates a small indentation in the posterior aspect of the sartorius muscle.

After the saphenous nerve leaves the adductor canal, it divides into the infrapatellar branch, which provides a sensory branch to the peripatellar plexus of the knee, and the sartorial branch, which perforates the superficial fascia between the gracilis and sartorius muscles, and emerges to lie in the subcutaneous tissue below the knee fold. It then descends along the medial tibial border with the long saphenous vein, giving multiple branches to the medial aspect of the leg, ankle, and forefoot. Ultrasound-guided infrapatellar nerve block can be performed, however, even with small volumes the saphenous nerve is blocked over 90% of the time.

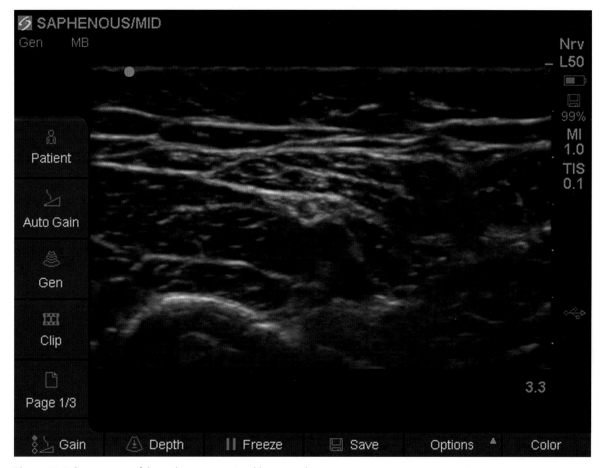

Figure 12.1 Sonoanatomy of the saphenous nerve in adductor canal.

Landmarks

Although ultrasound guidance allows visualization of the saphenous nerve throughout its course, three common sites are used:

1. Adductor canal
2. Just above the knee
3. Mid leg or above the ankle.

The child is placed supine.

To perform the adductor canal block, the ipsilateral hip is externally rotated with slight flexion of the knee. The probe is placed parallel to the inguinal ligament in the mid thigh region (Figure 12.3). For the mid leg or above the ankle approach, the child is positioned supine with the lower limb in neutral position.

Block performance

A high frequency linear probe is used for all three blocks.

Adductor canal block

The femoral artery is identified. One may continue scanning towards the knee following the femoral artery until the mid thigh where the femoral artery is usually found deep to the characteristically elliptical sartorius muscle.

Continue to scan caudally following the artery and nerve until the point of separation of the artery and nerve in order to avoid any accidental arterial puncture. The vastus medialis muscle will be anterolateral, the sartorius muscle will be medial and the adductor magnus muscle will lie posteromedial.

An in-plane approach is the commonest approach to allow visualization of the needle and its advancement (Figure 12.4). In younger children or neonates an out-of-plane approach may be needed to allow the shortest distance for needle advancement.

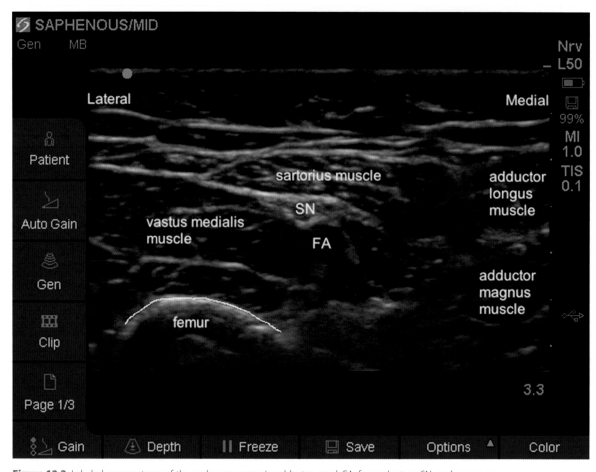

Figure 12.2 Labeled sonoanatomy of the saphenous nerve in adductor canal. FA, femoral artery; SN, saphenous nerve.

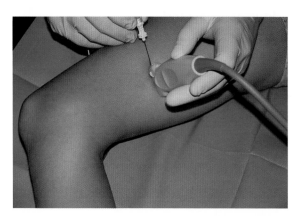

Figure 12.3 Patient position and probe placement for the adductor canal approach.

A 50-mm block needle may be used, and sufficient local anesthetic (LA) injected into the canal to surround the nerve. There are no data on the optimal dosing regime in children. A clinically effective volume is 0.2 ml/kg of bupivacaine 0.25% with epinephrine (1:200 000).

Just above the knee

This approach is mainly indicated for surgery of the medial aspect of the leg as an alternative to the mid-thigh approach. It has a lower risk of motor block, as the nerve to vastus medialis should have already separated. The probe is placed a few centimeters or 2–3 patient's own fingerbreadths above the patella on the anterior aspect. Following identification of the vastus medialis muscle, the probe is moved medially until the vastus medialis edge and the sartorius muscle is identified with its characteristic elliptical shape. By scanning the sartorius muscle a few centimeters cranially and caudally, the nerve can be identified as a small hyperechoic structure. This approach has the advantage of a lower incidence of arterial puncture.

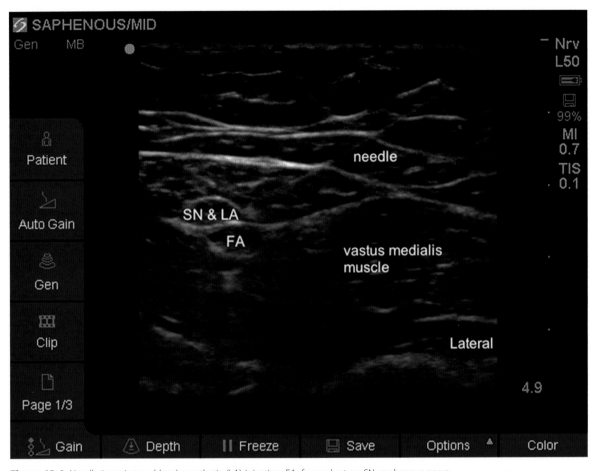

Figure 12.4 Needle insertion and local anesthetic (LA) injection. FA, femoral artery; SN, saphenous nerve.

Mid leg or above the ankle

This approach is beneficial for surgery on the foot, especially when combined with a popliteal block to provide complete analgesia to the foot. The key structure to identify is the saphenous vein as the nerve will be lying adjacent to it on either side. In children, the saphenous vein is very small and may be difficult to identify in addition to being easily compressible. Applying a tourniquet above the knee or allowing the knee to hang over the side of the trolley will allow congestion of the vein and may help with its identification alongside the use of color Doppler.

Post-operative care

The saphenous nerve block can be accompanied by some degree of quadriceps weakness as the nerve to vastus medialis muscle can be simultaneously blocked. Vigilance should be exercised during post-operative

mobilization of ambulatory patients. It is possible, but not common, to insert a catheter for continuous block of the saphenous nerve. Single shot injections, however, usually last for approximately 14–18 hours.

Clinical tips

- Ultrasound-guided saphenous nerve block is a relatively new technique.
- Quadriceps strength is maintained.
- The saphenous nerve can be blocked at a number of places along the inner thigh.
- The relationship of the nerve to the femoral artery changes, lying more distant to it as one travels distally.
- Hydro-dissection with LA placed between the vastus medialis and the sartorius muscles will improve visualization of this small nerve.

93

- A perivascular approach, with LA injected either side of the saphenous vein, can be used below the knee.
- Electrical stimulation may be used to differentiate the saphenous nerve (sensory) and the nerve to

vastus medialis muscle (motor stimulation) in the distal thigh.
- Motor blockade of the quadriceps should be assessed before mobilization.
- Complications are rare.

Suggested reading

Flack S, Anderson C. (2012) Ultrasound guided lower extremity blocks. *Paediatr Anaesth.* 22, 72–80.

Hebl J, Lennon R. (2010) *Mayo Clinic Atlas of Regional Anaesthesia and Ultrasound-Guided Nerve Blockade.* New York, NY: Oxford University Press.

Horn JL, Pitsch T, Salinas F, Benninger B. (2009) Anatomic basis to the ultrasound-guided approach for saphenous nerve blockade. *Reg Anaesth Pain Med.* 34,486–9.

Hunter LY, Louis DS, Riciardi JR, O'Connor GA. (1979) The saphenous nerve: its course and importance in medial arthrotomy. *Am J Sports Med.* 7,227–30.

Kent ML, Hackworth RJ, Riffenburgh RH, et al. (2013) A comparison of ultrasound-guided and landmark-based approaches to saphenous nerve blockade: a prospective, controlled, blinded, crossover trial. *Anesth Analg.* 117,265–70.

Kim DH, Lin Y, Goytizolo EA, et al. (2014) Adductor canal block versus femoral nerve block for total knee arthroplasty. *Anesthesiology.* 120,540–50.

Krombach J, Gray AT. (2007) Sonography for saphenous nerve block near the adductor canal. *Reg Anaesth Pain Med.* 32,369–70.

Manickam B, Perlas A, Duggan E, et al. (2009) Feasibility and efficacy of ultrasound-guided block of the saphenous nerve in the adductor canal. *Reg Anaesth Pain Med.* 34,578–80.

Peleritti H, Casalia AG. (2006) Internal saphenous nerve block. *Tech Reg Anesth Pain Manag.* 10,159–62.

Williams A, Newell R, Davis M, Collins P. (2005) Thigh. In Standing S, ed. *Gray's Anatomy: The Anatomical basis of Clinical Practice*, 39th edn. Philadelphia, PA: Elsevier–Churchill Livingstone.

Useful websites

www.jcrac.co.uk
www.nysora.com
www.usra.ca

Chapter

13

Ultrasound-guided sciatic nerve block

Anne-Charlotte Saour and Christophe Dadure

Clinical use

In children, lower limb surgery is commonly performed. The surgical correction of congenital orthopedic malformations is very painful as bony surgery is often required. The use of sciatic nerve block is common for post-operative analgesia after ankle or foot surgeries (arthrodesis or clubfoot repair) in pediatrics. In emergency surgery (ankle/foot fracture or amputation), it can be useful to combine sciatic nerve block with general anesthesia or sedation. However, care must be exercised in the use of peripheral nerve blockade in patients at risk of acute compartment syndrome (Mannion and Capdevila, 2010).

The sciatic nerve is a motor and sensory nerve consisting of the tibial and common peroneal nerves. It innervates the posterior aspect of the thigh and knee and all of the leg and foot except for the medial aspect of the calf and a small patch of skin between the first and second toes, which are innervated by the saphenous nerve. Subgluteal approaches to sciatic nerve blockade are useful for knee surgery, particularly if combined with complete or partial (saphenous nerve) blockade of the femoral nerve.

Ultrasound guidance expands the use of sciatic nerve block in pediatric regional anesthesia and allows for improvements in post-operative rehabilitation with continuous peripheral nerve catheters (Ponde et al., 2010; Van Geffen et al., 2010), especially in children with congenital orthopedic conditions (Ponde et al., 2013). Ultrasonography is able to visualize the sciatic nerve along its entire length and therefore blockade can be performed at a number of sites. The most common sites are the subgluteal and popliteal areas.

Ultrasound-guided sciatic nerve block improves success rates and prolongs the sensory blockade compared to traditional techniques (Oberndorfer et al., 2007).

Clinical sonoanatomy

The sciatic nerve arises from the sacral and lumbar plexus (fourth and fifth lumbar nerves join the first, second and third sacral nerves). It exits from the pelvis through the greater sciatic foramen, then descends between the great trochanter and ischial tuberosity until the apex of the popliteal fossa where it divides into two different nerves: the tibial nerve and the common peroneal nerve, which are contained within a common sheath (Figure 13.1). This site of the bifurcation is subject to significant anatomic variation (Schwemmer et al., 2004).

The sciatic nerve's whole length can be visualized sonographically, from the gluteal crease to its division in popliteal fossa. The nerve lies deep in the subgluteal region, becoming more superficial as it descends. The hyperechoic and oval structure of the sciatic nerve is located between the biceps femoris and the gluteus muscles at this level (Figure 13.2). The greater trochanter appears hypoechoic and lateral to the sciatic nerve.

Leaving the subgluteal region, the nerve runs between the long head of the biceps femoris (laterally) and the adductor magnus (medially) muscles initially. In the popliteal region the sciatic nerve is located between the biceps femoris laterally and the semi tendinous and semi membranous muscles medially. The popliteal artery runs medially and more superficial than the sciatic nerve and is of limited use in locating the nerve sonographically (Figure 13.1). It can, however, be used to locate the tibial nerve distally and then the tibial nerve can be followed cephalad to where it separates from the common peroneal nerve. The tibial nerve appears as a hyperechoic structure. The common peroneal nerve is smaller and more hypoechoic than tibial nerve, and runs more laterally.

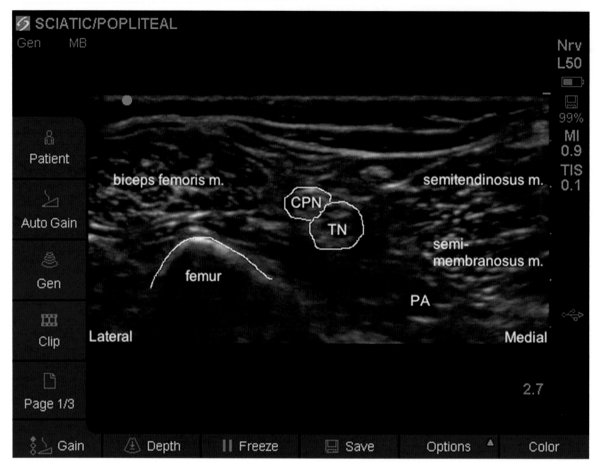

Figure 13.1 Sonoanatomy popliteal fossa. CPN, common peroneal nerve; TN, tibial nerve: both nerves constitute the sciatic nerve. PA, popliteal artery.

Landmarks

To visualize the sciatic nerve for the popliteal approach, the patient can be placed in the lateral, prone, or supine position. The supine position has advantages in children as positioning anesthetized patients in the prone or lateral positions may be difficult and may compromise the airway. In the supine position the probe must be positioned under the flexed knee and a lateral needle approach taken (Figure 13.3). In the prone or lateral positions the probe is placed in the region of the popliteal fossa and an in-plane or out-of-plane approach taken for needle insertion (Figure 13.4). A flexed knee in either position assists in identifying the muscle landmarks.

To visualize the sciatic nerve for the subgluteal approach, the patient can be placed in the lateral or prone position. The probe is then placed in the subgluteal region, below the cleft of the buttock (Figure 13.5).

Block performance

To perform either the subgluteal or the popliteal block, a linear high frequency probe is recommended. For older or obese children, a curved array probe can be required to perform the subgluteal block because of the deeper structures. In the infant population, the use of a "hockey-stick" probe is recommended (Ponde et al., 2013). Depending on the age of the child, the needle length is between 50 and 80 mm.

Popliteal block

For both the lateral and supine positions, the probe is placed transversally to the long axis of leg in the popliteal region. If the sciatic nerve is difficult to locate, the

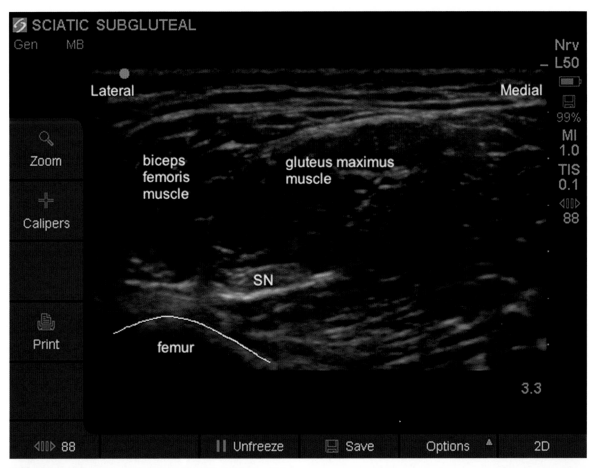

SCIATIC SUBGLUTEAL

Gen   MB

Lateral

biceps femoris muscle

gluteus maximus muscle

SN

femur

Nrv
– L50
99%
MI
1.0
TIS
0.1
88

Medial

Zoom

Calipers

Print

88   Unfreeze   Save   Options   2D

3.3

Figure 13.2 Sonoanatomy subgluteal region. SN, sciatic nerve.

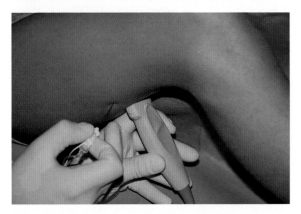

Figure 13.3 Probe placement for lateral popliteal block.

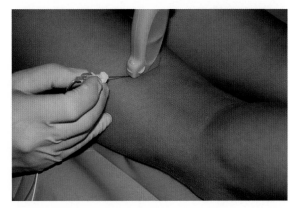

Figure 13.4 Probe placement for posterior popliteal block.

probe can be placed at the popliteal skin crease and the tibial nerve located because of its proximity to the popliteal artery. Then, the tibial nerve is followed by a cephalic movement of the probe until it converges with the common peroneal nerve to form the sciatic nerve.

If an in-plane needle approach is used, the needle is usually inserted through the lateral side of the thigh, between the vastus lateralis muscle and tendon of biceps femoris.

The orientation of the needle must be in line with the transverse probe position. The tip and shaft of

97

the needle must be visualized during the block performance until the targeted nerve is approached (Figure 13.6). The local anesthetic (LA) is injected around the sciatic nerve; the spread of the LA must

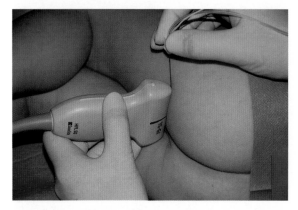

Figure 13.5 Probe placement for subgluteal approach for sciatic nerve block.

be seen as hypoechoic and ideally circumferential. The injection of LA may highlight the separate tibial and common peroneal components of the sciatic nerve and additional needle manipulation may be necessary to deposition sufficient LA around each nerve.

For insertion of a peripheral nerve catheter, some prefer to use an out-of-plane approach to insert the catheter more easily to the long axis of the nerve. This approach is not possible in the supine position as the needle tip is poorly seen or not visualized.

In the prone position, the leg to be blocked is raised so as to flex the knee. The probe is placed in the transverse position. In general the needle is introduced out-of-plane at 70 degrees to the skin.

The volume of LA usually injected is between 0.1–0.3 ml/kg of ropivacaine 0.2% or levobupivacaine 0.25% for prolonged blockade. Mepivacaine can be used for shorter neural blockade. For continuous sciatic nerve block, an infusion of 0.1 ml/kg/h of

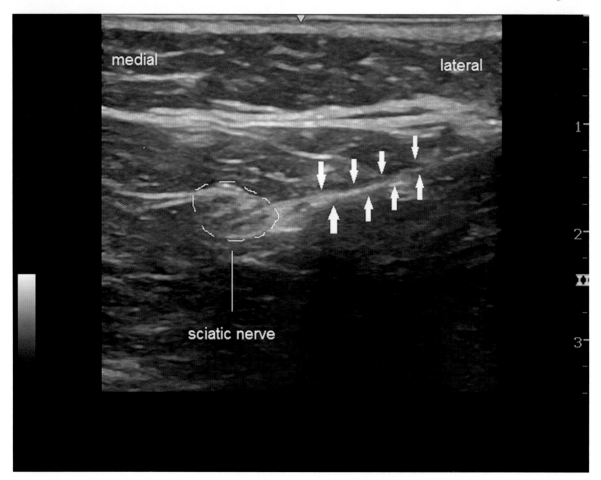

Figure 13.6 In-plane needle approach for lateral popliteal block. Needle is indicated by arrows.

0.1% or 0.2% ropivacaine (in infants or children respectively) is usually administered for 48–72 hours.

Subgluteal block

The probe is placed perpendicularly to the long axis of the thigh, and the sciatic nerve is scanned in a transverse plane (Gray et al., 2003). The hyperechoic and oval structure of the sciatic nerve is located between the biceps femoris and the gluteus muscles (Marhofer and Frickey, 2006; Roberts, 2006). Once the sciatic nerve is localized, the needle can be inserted out-of-plane or in-plane.

With the out-of-plane technique, the needle is inserted at 45 degrees to the skin, in the long axis of the nerve, perpendicular to the probe (Van Geffen et al., 2006). The needle progression is seen by a dorsal acoustic shadow emerging distal to the tip, or by the injection of a small volume of saline or LA. The technique of catheter insertion in the prone position was previously described by Van Geffen and colleagues (Van Geffen and Gielen, 2006; Van Geffen et al., 2010).

With an in-plane technique, the needle is inserted at 45 degrees to the skin. The needle is aligned to the long axis of the probe, allowing the visualization of the needle shaft and tip.

Post-operative care

Post-operative management is similar to other nerve blocks. A plan for post-operative analgesia must be in place both for rescue analgesia and the management of block resolution. Motor block should be monitored for, and the child allowed to mobilize only if assisted by at least one other person while motor blockade is present. Symptoms and signs of acute compartment syndrome must be monitored for, including removal or splitting of any casts. The presence of a cast can complicate diagnosis of whether neural signs or symptoms are block related or secondary to a compressive cast.

Clinical tips

- The sciatic nerve can be blocked using ultrasound guidance anywhere along its course in the thigh.
- The site of the division of the sciatic nerve into its tibial and common peroneal components is variable.
- For the popliteal approach, a supine position with lateral needle insertion avoids turning the child laterally or prone.
- The sciatic nerve can be more easily located by following the tibial nerve cephalad from the popliteal crease as it runs with the popliteal artery.
- The subgluteal approach allows placement of a catheter away from the surgery site in knee surgery.
- Mobilization of the patient should be assisted until full motor block resolution has occurred.

Suggested reading

Flack S, Anderson C. (2012) Ultrasound guided lower extremity blocks. *Paediatr Anaesth.* 22, 72–80.

Gray AT, Collins AB, Schafhalter-Zoppoth I. (2003) Sciatic nerve block in a child: a sonographic approach. *Anesth Analg.* 97,1300–2.

Mannion S, Capdevila X. (2010) Acute compartment syndrome and the role of regional anesthesia. *Int Anesthesiol Clin.* 48,85–105.

Marhofer P, Frickey N. (2006) Ultrasonographic guidance in pediatric regional anesthesia part 1: theoretical background. *Paediatr Anaesth.* 16,1008–18.

Oberndorfer U. Marhofer P, Bösenberg A, et al. (2007) Ultrasonographic guidance for sciatic and femoral nerve blocks in children. *Br J Anaesth.* 98,797–801.

Ponde V, Desai AP, Shah DM, Johari AN. (2010) Feasibility and efficacy of placement of continuous sciatic perineural catheters solely under ultrasound guidance in children: a descriptive study. *Paediatr Anaesth.* 21,406–10.

Ponde V, Desai AP, Shah DM. (2013) Comparison of success rate of ultrasound-guided sciatic and femoral nerve block and neurostimulation in children with arthrogryposis multiplex congenita: a randomized clinical trial. *Paediatr Anaesth.* 23,74–8.

Roberts S. (2006) Ultrasonographic guidance in pediatric regional anesthesia. Part 2: techniques. *Paediatr Anaesth.* 16,1112–24.

Schwemmer U, Markus CK, Greim CA, et al. (2004) Sonographic imaging of the sciatic nerve and its division in the popliteal fossa in children. *Paediatr Anaesth.* 14,1005–8.

Van Geffen G, Gielen M. (2006). Ultrasound-guided subgluteal sciatic nerve blocks with stimulating catheters in children: a descriptive study. *Anesth Analg.* 103, 328–33.

Van Geffen G., Scheuer M, Müller A, Garderniers J, Gielen M. (2006)

Ultrasound-guided bilateral continuous sciatic nerve blocks with stimulating catheters for postoperative pain relief after bilateral lower limb amputations. *Anaesthesia.* 61,1204–7.

Van Geffen G, Pirotte T, Gielen MJ, Scheffer G, Bruhn J. (2010). Ultrasound-guided proximal and distal sciatic nerve blocks in children. *J Clin Anesth.* 22, 241–5.

Chapter 14

Ultrasound-guided ilioinguinal/ iliohypogastric block

Sinead O'Shaughnessy and Charles Youngblood

Clinical uses

The ilioinguinal nerve is blocked in conjunction with the iliohypogastric nerve in the pediatric population to provide ipsilateral analgesia for inguinal and scrotal surgery. The technique is utilized for procedures including inguinal hernia repair, orchidopexy, or varicocelectomy. It is used as an analgesic adjunct to general anesthesia. The successful ilioinguinal/iliohypogastric block (ILIHB) provides long-lasting analgesia as well as reducing opioid consumption and opioid-related side effects. However, it is not sufficient to completely eliminate the visceral pain associated with peritoneal traction or manipulation of the spermatic cord or testes.

Developed in the 1980s, ILIHB was initially performed using anatomic landmarks and the "fascial click" method. However, a failure rate of up to 40% is reported with the landmark technique. This is mainly as a result of the high variability of pediatric anatomy, poorly defined landmarks, and intramuscular deposition of local anesthetic (LA). The introduction of ultrasound-guided techniques has achieved success rates of up to 95% and it is now regarded as the gold standard (Willschke et al., 2005). Ultrasound-guided ILIHBs also lower the dose required to achieve appropriate analgesia and reduce the complication rate. The use of lower doses of LA has particular relevance in neonates because of their increased risk of toxicity resulting from lower levels of alpha-1 acid glycoprotein (AAG) with subsequent reduced protein binding (Polaner and Drescher, 2011).

ILIHB can be as effective as the caudal block for post-operative analgesia and is accepted as a useful alternative (Markham at al., 1986). It has also been shown to establish superior levels of analgesia compared to the transversus abdominis plane (TAP) block for inguinal surgery (Bhalla et al., 2013).

ILIHB in children appears to be very safe. Overall, a complication rate of 1:1000 with no long-term consequences has been reported (Lönnqvist, 2010; Willschke at al., 2010). General complications include intravascular injection, infection, intraneural injection with subsequent nerve damage, and failure of the block to achieve the required analgesia. Specific complications are intraperitoneal injection, bowel perforation, hepatic injury, femoral nerve palsy, and pelvic hematoma. The distance between the deepest muscle layer, the transversus abdominis, and the bowel is minimal, further stressing the importance of an ultrasound-guided technique.

Clinical sonoanatomy

The ilioinguinal and iliohypogastric nerves are branches of the thoracolumbar plexus (T12/L1). The primary ventral ramus of L1 receives a branch from the twelfth spinal nerve and enters psoas major where it divides into the ilioinguinal and iliohypogastric nerves. Both emerge at the lateral border of psoas major, lying anterior to quadratus lumborum and posterior to the kidneys before piercing the lumbar fascia to run between transversus abdominis and internal oblique. The course of the iliohypogastric nerve is more superficial and superior to the ilioinguinal nerve, running between the internal oblique and external oblique before dividing into two terminal branches – the medial and lateral cutaneous nerves. The medial and lateral cutaneous nerves supply the lower abdominal wall and buttocks, respectively. The ilioinguinal nerve remains deep to the transversus abdominis until the level of the iliac crest where it becomes more superficial to supply the medial part of the thigh, the scrotum, and the base of the penis (van Schoor at al., 2005).

Ultrasound-Guided Regional Anesthesia in Children, ed. Mannion et al. Published by Cambridge University Press.
© Cambridge University Press 2015.

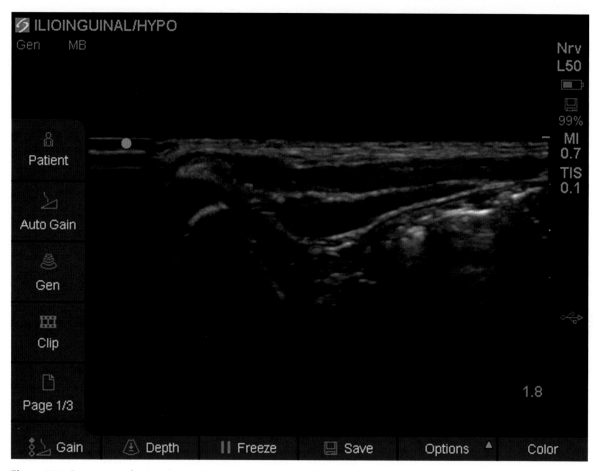

Figure 14.1 Sonoanatomy for the ilioinguinal/iliohypogastric block (ILIHB).

The main structures to visualize are the iliac crest laterally and the four tissue layers of the abdominal wall (Figure 14.1). These four layers comprise of adipose tissue, the external oblique, the internal oblique, and the transversus abdominis from superficial to deep. The peritoneum and intestines may be seen inferior to the transversus abdominis. In 50% of children, however, only two muscle layers are identified as the external oblique can be present solely as an aponeurosis. The ilioinguinal and iliohypogastric nerves can be identified as hyperechoic structures or hypoechoic with a hyperechoic rim, found in close proximity to the iliac crest. In this region these nerves may be found most commonly running in the plane between the internal oblique and the transversus abdominis muscles. They may, however, be seen separate; the iliohypogastric nerve lying between the external and internal obliques and the ilioinguinal nerve found between the internal oblique and the transversus abdominis muscles (Figure 14.2).

Landmarks

The child should be placed supine with the lower abdomen, iliac crest, and groin exposed. In order to identify the nerves, the probe is placed on the iliac crest along a line joining the anterior superior iliac spine (ASIS) with the umbilicus (Figure 14.3).

Identify all three muscle layers and the ilioinguinal/iliohypogastric nerves between the internal oblique and the transversus abdominis. Color Doppler will confirm the presence of any vascular structures in the same plane as the nerves.

Block performance

The block can be performed using an in-plane or out-of-plane approach using a 5–8 cm 22-gauge insulated needle. The in-plane approach confers the advantage of continuous assessment of needle position, which is important given the close proximity of the desired plane and the bowel (Weintraud at al., 2008). High-frequency

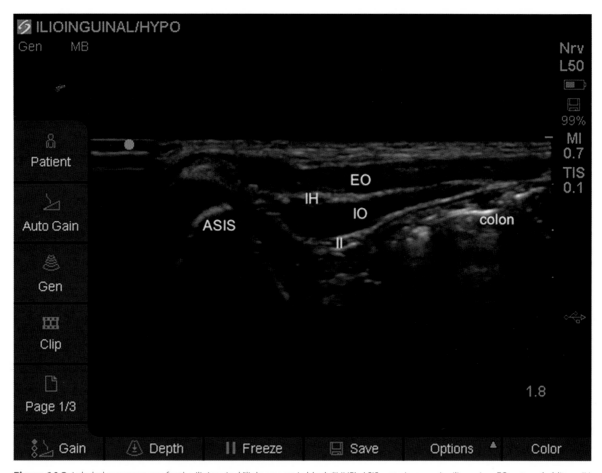

Figure 14.2 Labeled sonoanatomy for the ilioinguinal/iliohypogastric block (ILIHB). ASIS, anterior superior iliac spine; EO, external oblique; IH, iliohypogastric nerve; II, ilioinguinal nerve; IO, internal oblique.

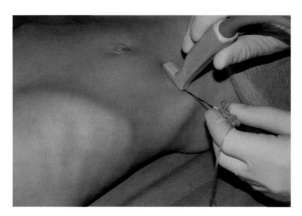

Figure 14.3 Patient position and probe placement. A lateral needle approach is performed.

linear ultrasound probes (5–10 MHz) can provide excellent definition as the nerves remain very superficial in the pediatric population, at a depth of approximately 1–3 cm. Bupivacaine 0.25% or levobupivacaine 0.25% are the most commonly used LA agents with a dose range of 0.1–0.2 ml/kg with a maximum volume of 10 ml. Doses as low as 0.075 ml/kg have previously been described with high success rates (Willschke at al., 2006).

Using an in-plane approach, the needle can be inserted either medially or laterally to the probe (Figure 14.4). The needle insertion point should be placed a short distance from the probe to allow visualization of the needle throughout the procedure.

Depending on the neural anatomy, two separate needle pathways may be required to deposit LA between the two oblique muscles or the internal oblique and transversus abdominis muscles only. Once the needle can be viewed in close proximity to the nerve (s) between the two muscle layers, careful aspiration is performed and a small volume of LA deposited. Once separation of the correct fascial layer is observed, the remaining LA can be injected. There are three principles of the correct injection technique. The first is to

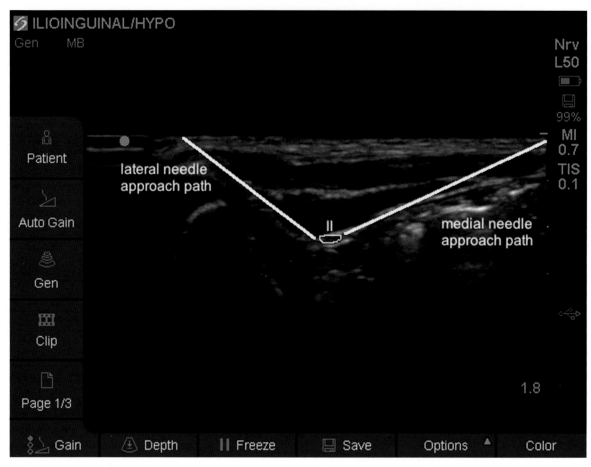

Figure 14.4 Needle pathway(s) and site of local anesthetic (LA) injection (outline) for block of ilioinguinal nerve (II).

locate the correct depth. This is achieved through needle visualization on ultrasound in conjunction with a "pop" or "fascial click" as the fascial layer is penetrated. The second principle states that minimal resistance should be encountered when injecting around the nerve, and the third principle is to never inject against resistance. The presence of resistance increases the likelihood that the needle tip is in muscle (Broen, 2012).

Alternatively an out-of-plane approach can be used. The needle is inserted at 90 degrees to the skin in the middle of the ultrasound screen. Progress of the needle causes tissue displacement, which allows assessment of needle tip position.

As no definitive method exists to identify LA toxicity, it is imperative that small doses are injected incrementally during the block. In addition, an observation period of up to 90 seconds after each dose has been suggested in order to detect any changes (Mosseti and Ivani, 2012).

Post-operative care

Post-operatively the patient should be observed for complications, initially in theater recovery and then on the pediatric ward. Supplementary analgesic requirements will confirm success of the block. Assessing ipsilateral power in the lower limb is important to rule out motor block secondary to spread of LA to the femoral nerve. Given this risk, we recommend bed rest or assisted mobilization for the duration of the block.

Clinical tips

- Ilioinguinal/iliohypogastric blocks are useful analgesic alternatives to caudal block for inguinal surgery.
- Use of ultrasound allows for lower doses of LA to be used and incurs fewer complications.

- Local anesthetic is placed between internal oblique and transversus abdominus superiorly to the anterior superior iliac spine.
- Use of in-plane technique is preferred to avoid peritoneal perforation.

- Rare complications include intraneural injection, intravascular injection, femoral nerve blockade, and bowel perforation.
- Intralipid® 20% should be immediately available when performing the block.

Suggested reading

Bhalla T, Sawardekar A, Dewhirst E, Jagannathan N, Tobias JD. (2013) Ultrasound-guided trunk and core blocks in infants and children. *J Anesth.* 27,109–23.

Bosenberg A. (2012) Regional anesthesia in children: the future. *Paediatr Anaesth.* 22, 564–9.

Broen TCK. (2012) History of pediatric regional anesthesia. *Paediatr Anaesth.* 22,3–9.

Lönnqvist P. (2010) Regional anaesthesia and analgesia in the neonate. *Best Pract Res Clin Anaesthesiol.* 24,309–21.

Markham SJ, Tomlinson J, Hain WR. (1986) Ilioinguinal nerve block in children. A comparison with caudal block for intra and postoperative analgesia. *Anaesthesia.* 41, 1098–103.

Mosseti V, Ivani G. (2012) Controversial issues in pediatric regional anaesthesia. *Paediatr Anaesth.* 22,109–14.

Polaner D, Drescher J. (2011) Paediatric regional anaesthesia: what is the current safety record? *Paediatr Anaesth.* 21,737–42.

Shah RD, Suresh S. (2013) Applications of regional anaesthesia in paediatrics. *Br J Anaesth.* 111,114–24.

van Schoor AN, Boon JM, Bosenberg AT, Abrahams PH, Meiring JH. (2005) Anatomical considerations of the pediatric ilioinguinal/iliohypogastric nerve block. *Paediatr Anaesth.* 15,371–7.

Weintraud M, Marhofer P, Bösenberg A, et al. (2008) Ilioinguinal/iliohypogastric blocks in children: where do we administer the local anesthetic without direct visualization? *Anesth Analg.* 106(1),89–93.

Willschke H, Marhofer P, Bösenberg A, et al. (2005). Ultrasonography for ilioinguinal/iliohypogastric nerve blocks in children. *Br J Anaesth.* 95 (2),226–30.

Willschke H, Bösenberg A, Marhofer P, et al. (2006). Ultrasonographic-guided ilioinguinal/iliohypogastric nerve block in pediatric anesthesia: what is the optimal volume? *Anesth Analg.* 102, 1680–4.

Willschke H, Marhofer P, Machata AM, Lönnqvist PA. (2010). Current trends in paediatric regional anaesthesia. *Anaesthesia,* 65, 97–104.

Chapter 15

Ultrasound-guided transversus abdominis plane block

Éimhín Dunne and Brian O'Donnell

Clinical use

The transversus abdominis plane (TAP) block is a somatic block of the abdominal wall. It has an established role in providing both intraoperative and post-operative analgesia for a wide range of abdominal surgery (McDonnell et al., 2007). The efficacy and safety of the TAP block in pediatric patients is less well described. For this reason, its use in the pediatric population remains limited, with central neuraxial blockade favored for post-operative analgesia in abdominal surgery (Mai et al, 2012). However, with increased recognition of the potential benefits of TAP blocks for pediatric patients, together with advancements in ultrasound technology, it has gained increasing popularity since the initial description in pediatric anesthesia in 2008 following inguinal hernia repair in 8 children (Fredrickson et al., 2008).

Originally described as the abdominal field block (Rafi, 2001), the landmark technique has undergone several modifications in an attempt to improve its analgesic efficacy. The term "transversus abdominis plane block" was coined in 2006 (McDonnell et al., 2007), a year before an ultrasound-guided technique was reported (Hebbard et al., 2007). Since then, further variations have been reported, with posterior, subcostal, and combined approaches all described. Considerable debate remains over which technique provides the best abdominal wall block for specific surgeries, with no particular approach being consistently superior in the available literature.

In contrast to the adult literature, few randomized studies have examined the efficacy and safety of the TAP block in pediatric patients. The lack of resources available to guide pediatric anesthetists likely explains the limited use of TAP blocks in this cohort of patients to date. Most information available to practicing clinicians

stems from published case reports and case series. However, a recently published safety analysis (Long et al., 2014) should lend confidence to clinicians and investigators performing this procedure, paving the way for more rigorous, larger randomized controlled trials.

Successful use of TAP blocks has been described for children spanning all age groups, including premature infants and neonates, with perioperative analgesic benefit for a wide array of surgical procedures including laparoscopy (diagnostic, appendicectomy, pyloromyotomy), laparotomy, umbilical surgery, formation and reversal of enterostomy/colostomy, open appendicectomy, inguinal hernia repair, hydrocelectomy, orchidopexy, scrotal exploration, and other abdominal wall surgery (closure exomphalos, closure gastroschisis, portosystemic shunt placement).

In addition, one case report demonstrated benefit in the management of hyperalgesia following abdominal surgery (Pak et al., 2009) and in chronic abdominal pain (Simpson et al., 2011) in pediatric patients.

Contraindications to TAP block are largely extrapolated from data on regional anesthesia techniques in the adult population. There is insufficient evidence to comment on coagulation status and whether or not it should be a relative contraindication to TAP block. This requires further investigation but the risk/benefit ratio should be determined on an individual case-by-case basis.

Only a few randomized trials examine the benefit of TAP blocks against other analgesic techniques. Fredrickson et al. randomly allocated 44 children aged between 6 months and 12 years presenting for elective inguinal surgery to receive TAP block or ilioinguinal nerve block, both performed under ultrasound guidance (Fredrickson et al., 2010). More children in the TAP block group (76% vs. 45%, $P = 0.04$) reported pain in the post-operative period and more required supplementary analgesia (62% vs. 30%, $P = 0.037$) when compared to the ilioinguinal nerve block group. As the authors acknowledge, the anatomic distribution of the most important nerves in inguinal surgery – the ilioinguinal, the iliohypogastric, and the genital branch of the genitofemoral nerve may be difficult to reach with the posterior approach to the TAP block chosen by the authors. However, they did report superior image quality and more efficient needle placement for the TAP block.

Sahin et al. compared ultrasound-guided TAP blocks with wound infiltration in 57 children aged between 2 and 8 years undergoing unilateral inguinal hernia repair (Sahin et al., 2013). The authors concluded that the high volume ultrasound-guided TAP block provided prolonged post-operative analgesia and reduced analgesic use.

Sandeman et al. prospectively randomized 93 children aged 7–16 years to receive ultrasound-guided TAP block or not in addition to wound infiltration for laparoscopic appendicectomy (Sandeman et al., 2011). Superior pain control was achieved in the first 6–8 hours of the post-operative period. However, overall morphine requirement in the first 16 hours after surgery was similar between the groups.

While there is currently insufficient evidence to recommend the use of TAP blocks over conventional techniques (Willschke and Kettner, 2012), there may be a role for using TAP block as part of a multimodal analgesic regime for certain procedures where central neuraxial blockade is contraindicated. Taylor et al. reported successful use of TAP catheters in two children with spinal dysraphism undergoing appendico-vesicostomy (Taylor et al., 2010). However, further randomized controlled trials are warranted to evaluate the efficacy and optimal dosing regime in the pediatric population.

A recent observational study estimated the overall complication rate of TAP block in the pediatric population at 0.3%. The study examined 1994 pediatric patients undergoing TAP block, 1887 of which were ultrasound-guided, and reported only 2 adverse events, neither of which warranted additional intervention (Long et al., 2014). One of the complications reported was positive aspiration of blood prior to injection of local anesthetic (LA), recognition of which prevented potentially more serious complications. The use of real-time ultrasonography facilitated recognition of the second complication – a peritoneal puncture – prior to further needle manipulation, which could

have potentially led to visceral puncture. It also allows the anesthesiologist to visualize the hypoechoic layer created by injection of LA in the TAP, confirming correct placement of the needle tip.

Further dose related considerations arise when extrapolating weight-based dosing from adults to the pediatric population. Optimal dosing may be influenced by reports suggesting that children's peripheral nerves may be more sensitive to LA when compared to adults (Benzon et al., 1998).

Clinical sonoanatomy

Ultrasound imaging of the anterior abdominal wall between the costal margin and the anterior superior iliac spine allows easy identification of the external oblique, the internal oblique, and the transversus abdominis muscles along with their associated hyperechoic fascial layer (Figure 15.1). Below the innermost muscle, the transversus abdominis, lies the transversalis fascia and the peritoneum (Figure 15.2).

The skin, muscles, and parietal peritoneum of the anterolateral abdominal wall are innervated by the anterior rami of lower six thoracic nerves (T7–T12) and first lumbar nerve (L1). The terminal branches of these nerves travel in the TAP between the internal oblique and transversus abdominis muscles.

The TAP block is a compartmental block targeting these nerves as they course through the anterolateral abdominal wall. Deposition of LA impairs nerve conduction resulting in sensory block of the anterolateral abdominal wall (skin and parietal peritoneum) (McDonnell et al., 2007). In clinical practice, the extent of the sensory block is variable, probably as a result of anatomic differences in nerve distribution and communication, technique used, site of needle insertion, and volume of LA injected.

Landmarks

Hebbard first described a *lateral approach* to the ultrasound-guided TAP block in adults (Hebbard, 2007). With the patient in the supine position, Hebbard recommended a transversely oriented probe on the anterolateral abdominal wall. Following identification of the TAP, the probe is moved posteriorly to the mid-axillary line, above the iliac crest. The needle tip is then directed posterior to the mid-axillary line prior to infiltration of LA, which can be visualized in real-time.

However, as this technique only reliably produced analgesia below the umbilicus, Hebbard went on to

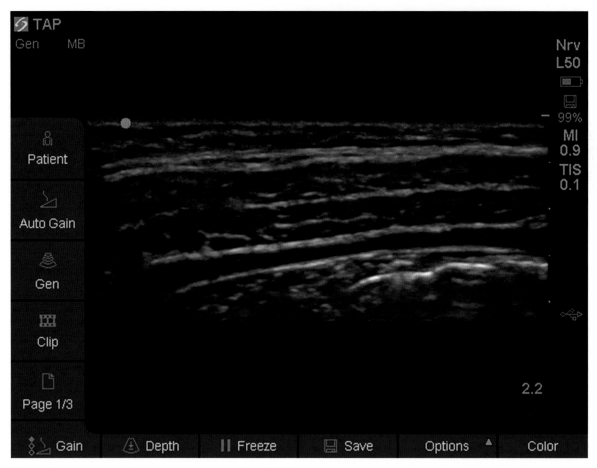

Figure 15.1 Sonoanatomy for transversus abdominis plane (TAP) block.

modify his approach to perform an "*oblique subcostal*" TAP block in 21 adult patients (Hebbard, 2008). He suggested placing the ultrasound probe perpendicular to the abdominal wall, parallel to the costal margin and oblique to the sagittal plane. The needle is introduced close to the xiphoid process in-plane with the probe, and LA is infiltrated between the transversus abdominis and rectus abdominis muscles. Hebbard then directed the needle infero-laterally to progressively distend the TAP. However, it must be pointed out that excessive needle movement potentially increases the risk of vascular and/or neural injury.

A further modification by Suresh and Chan was described in 2009 to overcome the difficulty in identifying the relevant sonoanatomy described by Hebbard in the oblique subcostal approach in newborns and infants (Suresh and Chan, 2009). The authors recommend placing a "hockey-stick" ultrasound transducer immediately lateral to the umbilicus to first identify the posterior rectal sheath and the rectus abdominis muscle. From that position, the probe is then moved laterally toward the flank where all three layers of the abdominal musculature are easily seen, becoming aponeurotic before the lateral border of latissimus dorsi and the origin of the transversus abdominis come into view. The reported benefit of this approach was to potentially allow for better spread of the drug to the entire abdominal wall as the local anesthetic was deposited closer to the origin of the thoracolumbar roots (Suresh and Chan, 2009).

Until further data in children are available, a reasonable site for injection is slightly posterior to the mid-axillary line with the probe position adjusted to obtain the best view of all three muscle layers (Figure 15.3). This *lateral* approach is described below. Upper abdominal incisions may be best served

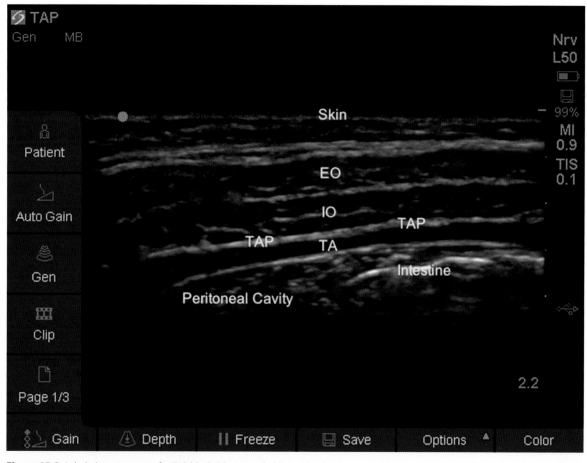

Figure 15.2 Labeled sonoanatomy for TAP block. EO, external oblique muscle; IO, internal oblique muscle; TA, transversus abdominis muscle; TAP, transversus abdominis plane.

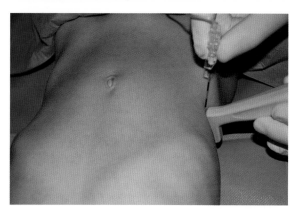

Figure 15.3 Patient position, probe placement, and in-plane needle approach.

by the oblique subcostal approach or a rectus sheath block at that level.

Data from the adult population suggest the posterior approach is more beneficial for surgery below the umbilicus, with the subcostal approach more suitable for upper abdominal incisions.

Block performance

For a posterior TAP block the transversely oriented probe is placed on the anterolateral abdominal wall between the costal margin and the iliac crest over the anterior axillary line (Figure 15.3). Once the three muscles of the anterior abdominal wall are identified, the probe is translated posteriorly to identify the origin of the transversus abdominis muscle, beneath the latissimus dorsalis muscle.

The needle is introduced in-plane at the medial aspect of the transducer in a medial to lateral orientation. A "pop" sensation may be appreciated as the needle passes through the plane between the external oblique and internal oblique, and again as it passes into the plane between the internal oblique and

109

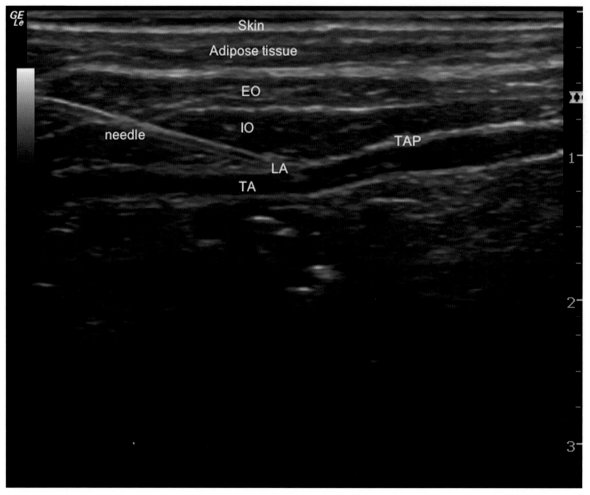

Figure 15.4 In-plane needle approach for TAP block. EO, external oblique muscle; IO, internal oblique muscle; LA, local anesthetic; TA, transversus abdominis muscle; TAP, transversus abdominis plane.

transversus abdominis muscle (Figure 15.4). Then, 1–2 ml of LA solution is injected to confirm correct location of the needle tip, which should appear hypoechoic on ultrasound. If the injection appears intramuscular, the needle tip is withdrawn or advanced by 1 or 2 mm before another aliquot of 1–2 ml is infiltrated to ensure location of the needle tip within the TAP. The drug of choice is a long-acting amide LA, such as bupivacaine 0.2% or ropivacaine 0.2%, and total LA dose should not exceed accepted safe maximal doses.

Current recommended doses for both bupivacaine and ropivacaine in children are 2 mg/kg. The addition of epinephrine to the LA solution may prolong analgesia and reduce peak plasma concentrations.

Post-operative care

The TAP block is a purely somatic block and will not provide analgesia for pain arising from visceral sources. As such, TAP should be considered as one component of a multimodal approach to postoperative pain management.

Clinical tips

- Placing LA posteriorly within transversus abdominis plane (TAP) appears to provide a more reliable analgesic result. It is thought that this is due to spread of LA along neural paths, over the quadratus lumborum muscle, and towards the paravertebral space.

- The deposition of LA within the TAP anteriorly or in the subcostal region results in limited abdominal wall block either below or above the umbilicus.
- Tilting the patient's pelvis laterally will permit access to the posterolateral abdominal wall. Use a small gel pad or pillow to achieve this tilt before commencing the block set-up.
- TAP block is a unilateral block. Midline incisions require a block on both sides of the abdomen.
- High serum levels of LA have been reported following TAP, and a recent report of seizures complicating TAP following a Cesarean section illustrate the potential for systemic toxicity (Weiss et al., 2014).
- Occasionally, quadriceps weakness has been reported following TAP. This is likely to be due to inadvertent femoral nerve block. If LA is deposited deep to the transversus muscle, it can track along the transversalis fascia, which is continuous with the fascia lata in the thigh. If this occurs, it is usually short-lived and no active remedy other than reassurance is required.

Suggested reading

Benzon HT, Strichartz GR, Gissen AJ et al. (1998) Developmental neurophysiology of mammalian peripheral nerves and age-related differential sensitivity to local anaesthetic. *Br J Anaesth.* 61,754–60.

Fredrickson M, Seal P, Houghton J. (2008) Early experience with the transversus abdominis plane block in children. *Paediatr Anaesth.* 18. 891–2.

Fredrickson MJ, Paine C, Hamill J. (2010) Improved analgesia with the ilioinguinal block compared to the transversus abdominis plane block after pediatric inguinal surgery: a prospective randomized trial. *Paediatr Anaesth.* 20,1022–7.

Hebbard P. (2008) Subcostal transversus abdominis plane block under ultrasound guidance. *Anesth Analg.* 106,674–5.

Hebbard P, Fujiwara Y, Shibata Y et al. (2007) Ultrasound-guided transversus abdominis plane (TAP) block. *Anaesth Intensive Care.* 35,616–17.

Long JB, Birmingham PK, De Oliveira GS, Schaldenbrand KM, Suresh S. (2014) Transversus abdominis plane block in children: a multicenter safety analysis of 1994 cases from the PRAN (Pediatric Regional Anesthesia Network) database. *Anesth Analg.* 119,395–9.

Mai CL, Young MJ, Quraishi SA. (2012) Clinical implications of the transversus abdominis plane block in pediatric anesthesia. *Paediatr Anaesth.* 22,831–42.

McDonnell JG, O Donnell B, Curley G et al. (2007) The analgesic efficacy of transversus abdominis plane block after abdominal surgery: a prospective randomized controlled trial. *Anesth Analg.* 104,193–7.

O'Donnell BD, McDonnell JG, McShane AJ. (2006) The transversus abdominis plane (TAP) block in open retropubic prostatectomy. *Reg Anesth Pain Med.* 31,91.

Pak T, Mickelson J, Yerkes E et al. (2009) Transverse abdominis plane block: a new approach to the management of secondary hyperalgesia following major abdominal surgery. *Paediatr Anaesth.* 19,54–6.

Palmer GM, Luk VHY, Smith KR et al. (2011) Audit of initial use of the ultrasound-guided transversus abdominis plane block in children. *Anaesth Intensive Care.* 39, 279–86.

Rafi AN. (2001) Abdominal field block: a new approach via the lumbar triangle. *Anaesthesia.* 56,1024–6.

Sahin L, Sahin M, Gul R, Saricicek V, Isikay N. (2013) Ultrasound-guided transversus abdominis plane block in children: a randomised comparison with wound infiltration. *Eur J Anaesthesiol.* 30,409–14.

Sandeman DJ, Bennett M, Dilley AV et al. (2011) Ultrasound-guided transversus abdominis plane blocks for laparoscopic appendicectomy in children: a prospective randomized trial. *Br J Anaesth.* 106,882–6.

Simpson DM, Tyrrell J, De Ruiter J et al (2011) Use of ultrasound-guided subcostal transversus abdominis plane blocks in a pediatric patient with chronic abdominal wall pain. *Paediatr Anaesth.* 21,88–90.

Suresh S, Chan VWS. (2009) Ultrasound guided transversus abdominis plane block in infants, children and adolescents: a simple procedural guidance for their performance. *Paediatr Anaesth.* 19,296–9.

Taylor LJ, Birmingham P, Yerkes E et al. (2010) Children with spinal dysraphism: transversus abdominis plane (TAP) catheters to the rescue! *Paediatr Anaesth.* 20,951–4.

Weiss E, Jolly C, Dumoulin L, et al. (2014) Convulsions in two patients after bilateral ultrasound-guided transversus abdominis plane blocks for Cesarean analgesia. *Reg Anesth Pain Med.* 39(3),248–51.

Willschke H, Kettner S. (2012) Pediatric regional anesthesia: abdominal wall blocks. *Paediatr Anaesth.* 22,88–92.

Chapter

16

Ultrasound-guided rectus sheath block

Harshad Gurnaney and Arjunan Ganesh

Clinical use

The rectus sheath block can be used to provide postoperative analgesia for anterior abdominal procedures (Gurnaney et al., 2011). In 1996 the rectus sheath block was suggested as an option for providing postoperative analgesia for an umbilical hernia repair (Ferguson et al., 1996). Since then this technique has been used to provide analgesia for umbilical and epigastric hernia repair, laparoscopic surgery, and other small midline incisions and has been found to provide better analgesia than wound infiltration (Breschan et al., 2013; Dingeman et al., 2013; Flack et al., 2014). It has also been used for the relief of chronic abdominal wall pain (Skinner and Lauder, 2007). A rectus sheath catheter technique can be used for midline laparotomy procedures for providing postoperative analgesia (Courreges and Poddevin, 1998).

The rectus sheath block anesthetizes the anterior divisions of the seventh, eighth, ninth, tenth, and eleventh thoracic intercostal nerves, which are called the thoracoabdominal nerves. These nerves innervate the anterior abdominal wall. They continue anteriorly from the intercostal space into the abdominal wall. In the abdominal wall the nerves reach the posterior layer of the internal oblique aponeurosis and continue between the transversus abdominis and internal oblique muscles. At the lateral border of the rectus abdominis muscle, the external oblique aponeurosis and the anterior lamella of the internal oblique aponeurosis form the anterior rectus sheath, while the posterior lamella of the internal oblique aponeurosis and the aponeurosis of the transversus abdominis form the posterior rectus sheath. At the lateral edge of the rectus abdominis muscle each nerve pierces the internal oblique aponeurosis and lies between the rectus abdominis muscle and the posterior rectus sheath. These nerves supply the rectus abdominis and end as the anterior cutaneous branch of the abdomen. The ninth thoracic nerve supplies the skin above the umbilicus, the tenth nerve supplies the umbilical region, and the eleventh nerve supplies the skin below the umbilicus.

This region is readily visualized using ultrasound, allowing accurate deposition of local anesthetic (LA) into the rectus sheath itself (Flack et al., 2014). No correlation has been found between the depth of the posterior rectus sheath and the child's weight, height, or body surface area (Willschke et al., 2006).

Clinical sonoanatomy

The rectus abdominis muscle is visualized as an oval-shaped muscle in the anterior abdominal wall (Figure 16.1). The anterior and posterior rectus sheaths are visualized and can be followed laterally, where they become the aponeurosis of the external oblique, the internal oblique, and the transversus abdominis muscles. The ninth, tenth, and eleventh intercostal nerves lie between the rectus abdominis muscle and the posterior rectus sheath. These nerves are difficult to identify in this location using ultrasound, but the posterior rectus sheath and the rectus abdominis muscle can be easily identified (Figure 16.2). It is important to remember that the superior epigastric vessels (artery and vein) also travel in the same plane or within the body of the rectus abdominis muscle. Color Doppler can be used to identify the vessels if hypoechoic structures are found in this location. Deep to the posterior rectus sheath is the peritoneum and the intraperitoneal content (stomach and intestines).

Ultrasound-Guided Regional Anesthesia in Children, ed. Mannion et al. Published by Cambridge University Press.
© Cambridge University Press 2015.

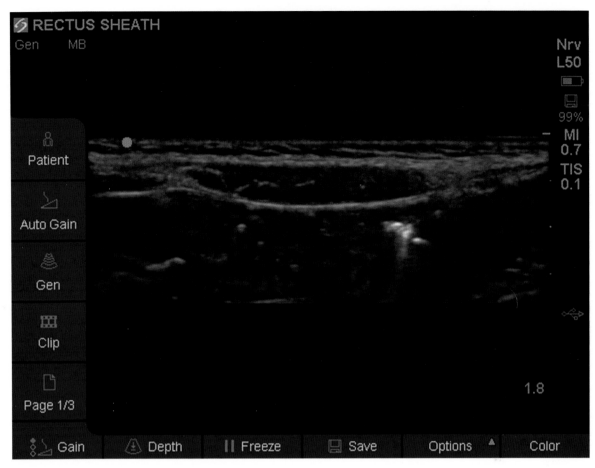

Figure 16.1 Sonoanatomy for a rectus sheath block.

Landmarks

The child is placed supine and the outline of the rectus muscle sheath is determined by palpation or ultrasound imaging. The rectus muscles are usually easy to palpate along their length in small children. The probe is placed at the appropriate level, bearing in mind that a number of injections may be required depending on the extent of surgery (Figure 16.3). Bilateral blocks are required for any midline surgeries.

Block performance

In children a high-frequency low penetrance probe may be sufficient for visualization of the rectus muscle and sheath in the anterior abdominal wall. The depth of the rectus muscle can be variable depending on the amount of subcutaneous tissue. The ultrasound probe can be scanned laterally to identify the junction of the external oblique, internal oblique, and transversus abdominis muscles with the

rectus abdominis muscle. The epigastric vessels should also be identified.

The needle is inserted in-plane in a lateral to medial direction and advanced through the anterior rectus sheath and the rectus abdominis muscle. The needle is advanced until the tip is through the muscle and lying on the posterior rectus sheath (Figure 16.4). A small amount of LA or saline can be used to confirm that the location of the needle tip is not intramuscular prior to injection of the appropriate dose of LA.

For single injection a 22-gauge 50 mm short-bevel needle can be used, and the length of needle can be elected based on child size and depth of the rectus sheath.

A volume of 0.1 ml/kg of 0.25% bupivacaine or 0.2% ropivacaine is recommended for a rectus sheath block (Flack et al., 2014).

The same procedure should be repeated on the opposite side. An out-of-plane technique may also be used to perform a rectus sheath block.

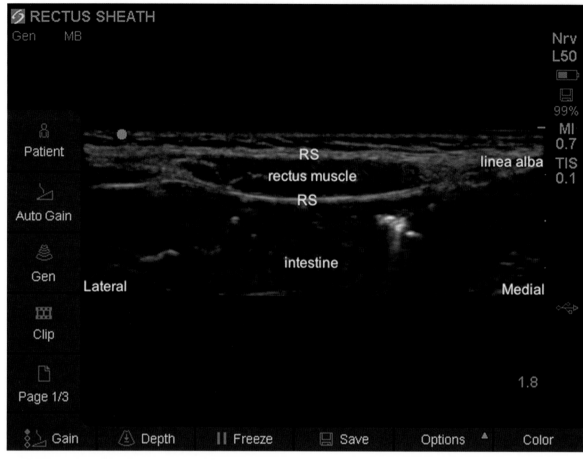

Figure 16.2 Labeled sonoanatomy for a rectus sheath (RS) block.

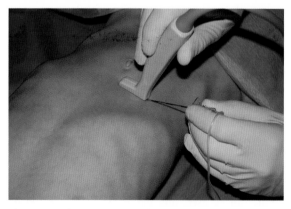

Figure 16.3 Patient position and probe placement for umbilical surgery.

Continuous catheter technique

The patient position and probe orientation are similar to that of a single injection technique. Once the needle tip is positioned between the rectus abdominis muscle and the posterior rectus sheath, 1–2 ml of normal saline can be injected to confirm the tip location. This will also ease the advancement of the catheter into the space between the rectus abdominis muscle and the posterior rectus sheath. Once the catheter is inserted, the catheter tip position is confirmed by visualizing an injection of a small amount of LA through the catheter. Following this confirmation, the intended dose of LA is administered through the catheter.

Post-operative care

Most patients with single shot blocks can be discharged home prior to resolution of the block. It is important to prepare the child's parents for the eventual resolution of the block and the potential for increased pain and anxiety in the child while he or she is at home. A plan for oral analgesics should be available and reviewed with the family prior to discharge.

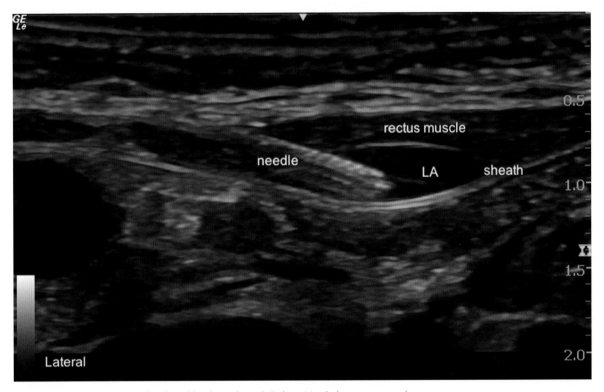

Figure 16.4 Needle in rectus sheath and local anesthetic (LA) deposition below rectus muscle.

Clinical tips

- Ultrasound examination of the relevant anatomy should be undertaken prior to performing this block.
- As the needle tip is being advanced through the belly of the rectus abdominis muscle a small amount of normal saline can be injected to confirm the needle tip location between the rectus abdomis and the posterior rectus sheath, which is visualized as the muscle belly being separated from the posterior rectus sheath.
- Bilateral blocks are required for midline surgeries.
- A number of blocks at different levels may be required for extensive surgery.

Suggested reading

Breschan C, Jost R, Stettner H, et al. (2013) Ultrasound-guided rectus sheath block for pyloromyotomy in infants: a retrospective analysis of a case series. *Paediatr Anaesth.* 23,1199–204.

Courreges P, Poddevin F. (1998) Rectus sheath block in infants: what suitability? *Paediatr Anaesth.* 8,181–2.

Dingeman RS, Barus LM, Chung HK, et al. (2013) Ultrasonography-guided bilateral rectus sheath block vs. local anesthetic infiltration after pediatric umbilical hernia repair: a prospective randomized clinical trial. *JAMA Surg.* 148,707–13.

Dolan J, Smith M. (2009) Visualization of bowel adherent to the peritoneum before rectus sheath block: another indication for the use of ultrasound in regional anesthesia. *Reg Anesth Pain Med.* 34,280–1.

Ferguson S, Thomas V, Lewis I. (1996) The rectus sheath block in paediatric anaesthesia: new indications for an old technique? *Paediatr Anaesth.* 6,463–6.

Flack SH, Martin LD, Walker BJ, et al. (2014) Ultrasound-guided rectus sheath block or wound infiltration in children: a randomized blinded study of analgesia and bupivacaine absorption. *Paediatr Anaesth.* 24,968–73.

Gurnaney HG, Maxwell LG, Kraemer FW, et al. (2011) Prospective randomized observer-blinded study comparing the analgesic efficacy of ultrasound-guided rectus sheath block and local anaesthetic infiltration for umbilical hernia repair. *Br J Anaesth.* 107,790–5.

Skinner AV, Lauder GR. (2007) Rectus sheath block: successful use in the chronic pain management of pediatric abdominal wall pain. *Paediatr Anaesth.* 17,1203–11.

Willschke H, Bösenberg A, Marhofer P, et al. (2006) Ultrasonography-guided rectus sheath block in paediatric anaesthesia-a new approach to an old technique. *Br J Anaesth.* 97,244–9.

Yuen PM, Ng PS. (2004) Retroperitoneal hematoma after a rectus sheath block. *J Am Assoc Gynecol Laparosc.* 11,448.

Chapter

17

Ultrasound-guided paravertebral block

Attila Bondár and Gabriella Iohom

Clinical use

The paravertebral block was first described in 1905 by Hugo Sellheim in an attempt to find an alternative to spinal anesthesia. This new approach, which targeted the spinal nerves at the emergence from the spinal column, was found to be safer than spinal anesthesia, having less adverse cardiovascular effects. However, the technique was largely abandoned until 1979, when Eason and Wyatt reintroduced the paravertebral block into modern-day regional anesthesia practice (Eason and Wyatt, 1979).

Paravertebral blocks can provide excellent postoperative analgesia in children for thoracic and abdominal procedures. Both unilateral single injection blocks (thoracoscopy, renal surgery, inguinal hernia) and bilateral single injection blocks (small umbilical hernia) have been described. While the efficacy of single injection blocks is limited (Hill et al., 2006), the insertion of a catheter can prolong post-operative analgesia up to several days (Boretsky et al., 2013). Unilateral continuous blocks are commonly performed for thoracoscopy, thoracotomy, rib resection, rib fractures, thoracoscopic aortopexy, patent ductus arteriosus ligation, abdominal wall mass excision, and renal surgery. Bilateral continuous blocks are also performed for laparotomy, bowel resection, Wilms tumor resection, pancreatectomy, and splenectomy (Visoiu and Yang, 2011; Ali and Akbar, 2013; Boretsky et al., 2013). Paravertebral blocks may have a role in the management of chronic pain in children.

Paravertebral blocks are associated with a high success rate, while placement of a thoracic epidural is often difficult and is associated with frequent failure (Chelly, 2012). Compared to thoracic epidurals, patients having paravertebral blocks experience less hypotension (especially if unilateral), no urinary retention, no motor weakness, and no opioid-related side effects; they also need less nursing resources and less monitoring (Pintaric et al., 2011). Serious complications related to epidurals, such as spinal haematoma and spinal cord injury, can be avoided. Paravertebral blocks (bilateral continuous) were successfully used in a mildly coagulopathic child, where the use of a thoracic epidural would have been strictly contraindicated (Visoiu and Yang, 2011). Advantages of ultrasound guidance over landmark-based and nerve stimulator techniques include: higher success rate, reduced local anesthetic (LA) volumes, and decreased time of block performance.

Overall incidence of complications of the paravertebral blocks in children were rare (Lönnqvist et al., 1995; Naja and Lönnqvist, 2001; Berta et al., 2008), even before the introduction of the ultrasound techniques. Complications may include: inadvertent pleural puncture, pneumothorax, vascular puncture, paravertebral hematoma, hypotension, contralateral paravertebral, epidural or intrathecal spread, neural injury, LA systemic toxicity, and failure. In the adult population there have been case reports of ipsilateral brachial plexus block, phrenic nerve paresis, Horner's syndrome (Renes et al., 2011) and Harlequin syndrome (Burlacu and Buggy, 2005). Performing the paravertebral block under direct vision using ultrasound guidance is likely to further reduce the rate of complications and improve success rates, although does not entirely eliminate complications. One small study using ultrasound guidance for catheter insertion in infants and children, showed no clinical evidence of complications or adverse effects (Boretsky et al., 2013).

Contraindications include patient/parent refusal, puncture site infection (dermatitis, psoriasis), empyema, tumor occupying the paravertebral space, coagulation disorder (relative contraindication), and undiagnosed or undocumented neurologic condition at the block level. Kyphoscoliosis and previous thoracotomy scarring can cause difficulty in locating the paravertebral space and can hinder local anesthetic spread (Gerard and Roberts, 2012).

Clinical sonoanatomy

The wedge-shaped paravertebral space can be found on either side of the spinal column (Figure 17.1). It extends from the cervical region to the psoas muscle. It is bounded antero-laterally by the endothoracic fascia and the parietal pleura, posteriorly by the anterior aspect of the transverse process and the superior costotransverse ligament, which is continuous with the internal intercostal membrane, and medially by the posterolateral aspect of the vertebral body, the intervertebral disc and foramen. Spinal

nerves exit the dural sleeve at the intervertebral foramen and travel through the paravertebral space to enter the intercostal space becoming intercostal nerves, and later thoracoabdominal nerves. Traditionally, the paravertebral space was identified using the landmark-based loss-of-resistance (Richardson and Lönnqvist, 1998) or the nerve stimulator technique (Lang, 2002). With the advent of ultrasound several new techniques have been described using real-time guidance in adults: the sagittal paramedian in-plane approach (Bondár et al., 2010; O'Riain et al., 2010), the lateral out-of-plane approach (Marhofer et al., 2010), the lateral in-plane approach (Renes et al., 2010), and, in cadavers, the intercostal in-plane approach (Ben-Ari et al., 2009), the oblique in-plane approach (Luyet et al., 2009). Some authors developed formulae for pediatric paravertebral blocks using computed tomography (CT) guidance (Yoo et al., 2012) and ultrasound guidance (Ponde and Desai, 2012) to estimate the appropriate depth and distance.

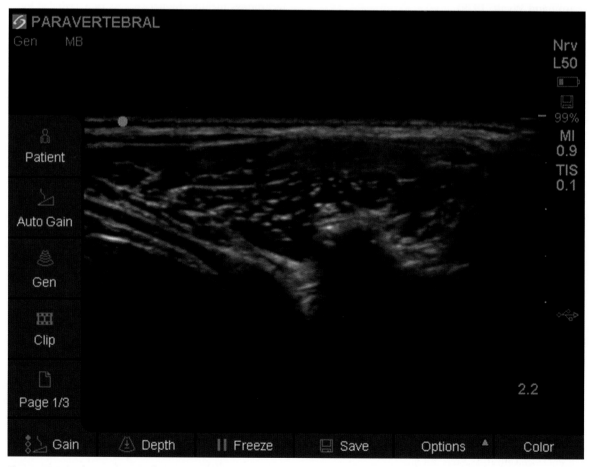

Figure 17.1 Axial sonoanatomy of the paravertebral space.

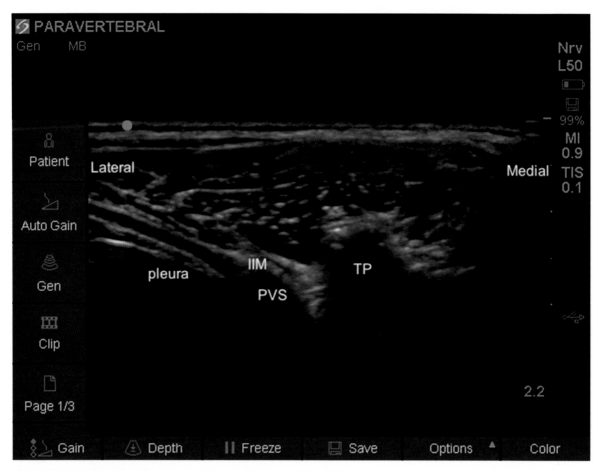

Figure 17.2 Labeled axial sonoanatomy of the paravertebral space (PVS). IIM, internal intercostal membrane; TP, transverse process.

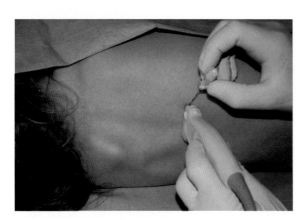

Figure 17.3 Lateral patient position and probe placement.

Since no pediatric guidelines for paravertebral block exist, the lateral in-plane and the sagittal paramedian approaches have been performed preferntially by pediatric anesthesiologists. In the latter approach, the steep insertion angle necessary to enter the space

between adjacent transverse processes makes continuous needle visualization difficult or impossible. Considering the reduced depth and distances and close proximity of vital structures, this technique is regarded as hazardous by some anesthesiologists (Boretsky et al., 2013). In the lateral in-plane approach the ultrasound probe is placed in the transverse paramedian position to obtain a clear visualization of the transverse process, the parietal pleura, the erector spinae muscle, the internal intercostal membrane, and the paravertebral space (Figure 17.2).

Landmarks

For unilateral paravertebral block the patient is placed in the lateral position with the operative side uppermost (Figure 17.3). For bilateral blocks the child is positioned either in prone position or in lateral position with the shoulder tilted forward forming a 45 degree angle with the bed to allow easy access to

119

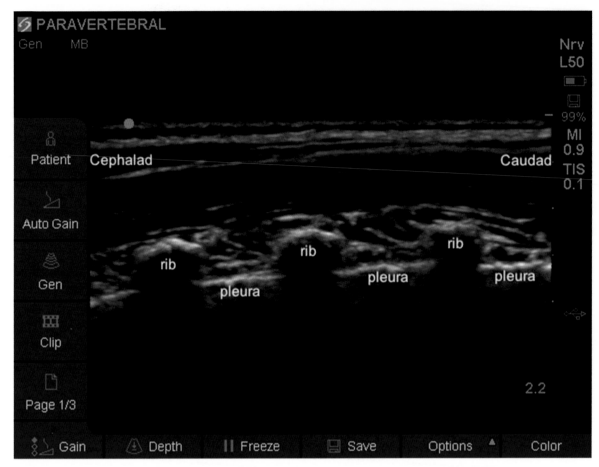

Figure 17.4 Labeled sagittal sonoanatomy of the paravertebral space. The probe has been moved slightly lateral to the midline to reveal the ribs and the relevant level. The pleural depth can be easily measured.

both sides of the back. The bed can be further tilted to optimize block performance (Boretsky et al., 2013). The appropriate vertebral level – T5 for thoracic procedures and T10 for abdominal surgeries – is identified either with the surface landmarks or using ultrasound to give a sagittal view (Figure 17.4), and marked. The ultrasound probe is placed over the marked spinous process in the midline and rotated perpendicular to the spinal column. Then, the probe is moved laterally to obtain an axial or transverse view of the transverse process and the parietal pleura (transverse paramedian view) (Figure 17.3). Probe tilting, rotation, and/or slide may be necessary to obtain a clear view of the important structures.

Block performance

In the pediatric population, a high frequency linear probe (>10 MHz) is appropriate, although some advocate a probe configuration based on age, weight, and body mass index (Boretsky et al., 2013). The ultrasound probe is positioned and manipulated until a clear image of the transverse process, the parietal pleura, and the internal intercostal membrane (lateral continuation of the costotransverse ligament) is obtained. Using an in-plane approach from lateral to medial, an appropriately sized Tuohy needle is introduced 1–2 cm from the lateral edge of the probe. The needle is advanced carefully under constant direct vision until the tip of the needle pierces the internal intercostal membrane and enters the paravertebral space (Figure 17.5). Correct position of the needle tip can be confirmed by resistance-free injection of 1 or 2 ml of normal saline and anterior displacement of the parietal pleura. After negative aspiration the LA can be injected and/or the catheter inserted. When placing a catheter, the bevel of the Tuohy needle should be oriented cranially in order to direct the

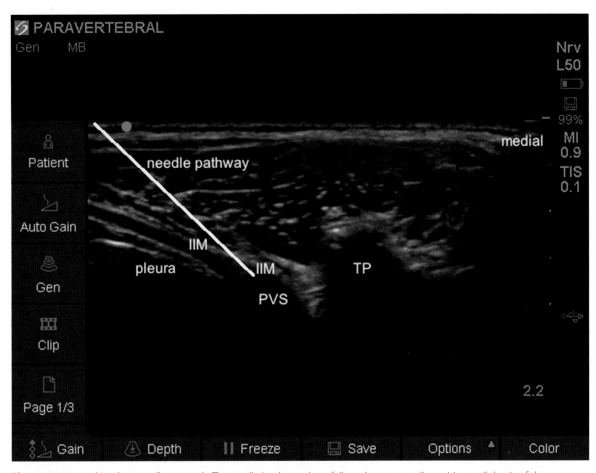

Figure 17.5 Lateral in-plane needle approach. The needle is advanced carefully under constant direct vision until the tip of the needle pierces the internal intercostal membrane and enters the paravertebral space (PVS). IIM, internal intercostal membrane; TP, transverse process

catheter in the cephalad direction. Catheters should be inserted no more than 2–3 cm beyond the needle tip, and correct catheter position is confirmed with additional anterior displacement of the parietal pleura following normal saline administration. Catheters may be tunneled. Although, the only pediatric study using ultrasound for catheter placement reported no catheter malfunction (Boretsky et al., 2013), adult cadaver studies suggest a high incidence of catheter misplacement into the epidural, mediastinal, or pleural spaces (Luyet et al., 2009, 2011). The optimal volume of LA in a single injection was suggested as 0.5 ml/kg per side (Lönnqvist and Hesser, 1993), which covers at least 5 thoracic paravertebral segments. However, a recent pediatric cadaver study shows that smaller volumes of 0.2 and 0.3 ml/kg are sufficient to cover 5 and 6 segments, respectively (Albokrinov and Fesenko, 2014). When a catheter is

placed, an infusion rate of 0.5 mg/kg/h is appropriate. LAs administered are: levobupivacaine 0.25%, bupivacaine 0.25%, or lidocaine 1% – all with added epinephrine 1:200 000 (Coté et al., 2013); ropivacaine 0.5% intraoperatively and 0.1% or 0.2% postoperatively (Boretsky et al., 2013).

Post-operative care

Since the effect of a single injection paravertebral block lasts up to 8 hours, oral and/or intravenous analgesics need to be prescribed and the paravertebral block should be considered as part of a multimodal analgesia regimen. When a catheter is placed, the LA infusion is started either in the operating room or in the postanesthesia care unit (PACU) according to local protocols. Post-operative pain should be assessed regularly using either the FLACC scale (Merkel, 1997) or the numeric rating score (NRS), and managd accordingly. A recent study shows that ambulatory continuous paravertebral nerve block is feasible for pediatric patients (Visoiu et al., 2014).

filled tubing and syringe to the needle while advancing the needle. In case of an inadvertent pleural puncture it prevents conversion to pneumothorax.

Clinical tips

- Use ultrasound guidance.
- Use an in-plane approach to visualize needle advancement and needle tip. Connect a fluid-

- Thread the catheter no more than 2–3 cm beyond the needle tip.
- Use normal saline for hydrodissection and identification of the paravertebral space in order to reduce the total LA dose administered.

Suggested reading

Albokrinov AA, Fesenko UA. (2014). Spread of dye after single thoracolumbar paravertebral injection in infants. A cadaveric study. *Eur J Anaesthesiol.* 31,305–9.

Ali MA, Akbar AS. (2013) Report of a case of ultrasound guided continuous thoracic paravertebral block for post thoracotomy analgesia in a child. *Middle East J Anesthesiol.* 22,107–8.

Ben-Ari A, Moreno M, Chelly JE, et al.. (2009) Ultrasound-guided paravertebral block using an intercostal approach. *Anesth Analg.* 109,1691–4.

Berta E, Spanhel J, Smakal O, et al. (2008) Single injection paravertebral block for renal surgery in children. *Paediatr Anaesth.* 18,593–7.

Bhalla T, Sawardekar A, Dewhirst E, et al. (2013) Ultrasound-guided trunk and core blocks in infants and children. *J Anesth.* 27,109–23.

Bondár A, Szűcs S, Iohom G. (2010) Thoracic paravertebral blockade. *Med Ultrason.* 12,223–7.

Boretsky K, Visoiu M, Bigeleisen P. (2013) Ultrasound-guided approach to the paravertebral space for catheter insertion in infants and children. *Paediatr Anaesth.* 23,1193–8.

Burlacu CL, Buggy DJ. (2005) Coexisting Harlequin and Horner syndromes after high thoracic paravertebral anaesthesia. *Br J Anaesth.* 95,822–4.

Chelly JE. (2012) Paravertebral blocks. *Anesthesiol Clin.* 30,75–90.

Coté CJ, Lerman J, Anderson BJ. (2013) *A Practice of Anesthesia for Infants and Children*, 5th edn. Philadelphia, PA: Elsevier Saunders.

Eason MJ, Wyatt R. (1979) Paravertebral thoracic block – a reappraisal. *Anaesthesia.* 34, 638–42.

Gerard C, Roberts S. (2012) Ultrasound-guided regional anaesthesia in the paediatric population. *ISRN Anesthesiology.* Article ID 169043.

Hill SE, Keller RA, Stafford-Smith M. et al. (2006) Efficacy of singe-dose, multilevel paravertebral nerve blockade for analgesia after thoracoscopic procedures. *Anesthesiology.* 104,1047–53.

Lang SA. (2002) The use of a nerve stimulator for thoracic paravertebral block. *Anesthesiology.* 97,521.

Lönnqvist PA, Hesser U. (1993) Radiological and clinical distribution of thoracic paravertebral blockade in infants and children. *Paediatr Anaesth.* 3,83–7.

Lönnqvist PA, MacKenzie J, Soni AK, et al. (1995) Paravertebral blockade. Failure rate and complications. *Anaesthesia.* 50,813–15.

Luyet C, Eichenberger U, Greif R. et al. (2009) Ultrasound-guided thoracic paravertebral puncture and placement of catheters in human

cadavers: an imaging study. *Br J Anaesth.* 102,534–9.

Luyet C, Herrmann G, Ross S. et al. (2011) Ultrasound-guided thoracic paravertebral puncture and placement of catheters in human cadavers: where do catheters go? *Br J Anaesth.* 106,246–54.

Marhofer P, Kettner SC, Hajbok L, et al. (2010) Lateral ultrasound-guided paravertebral blockade: an anatomical-based description of a new technique. *Br J Anaesth.* 105,526–32.

Merkel S. (1997) The FLACC: a behavioral scale for scoring postoperative pain in young children. *Pediatr Nurse.* 23,293–7.

Naja MZ, Lönnqvist PA. (2001) Somatic paravertebral nerve blockade: incidence of failed block and complications. *Anaesthesia.* 56,1184–8.

O'Riain SC, Donnell BO, Cuffe T, et al. (2010) Thoracic paravertebral block using real-time ultrasound guidance. *Anesth Analg.* 110,248–51.

Pintaric TS, Potocnik I, Hadzic A, et al. (2011) Comparison of continuous thoracic epidural with paravertebral block on perioperative analgesia and hemodynamic stability in patients having open lung surgery. *Reg Anesth Pain Med.* 36,256–60.

Ponde VC, Desai AP. (2012) Echo-guided estimation of formula for paravertebral block in neonates, infants and children till 5 years. *Indian J Anaesth.* 56,382–6.

Renes SH, Bruhn J, Gielen MJ, et al. (2010) In-plane ultrasound-guided thoracic paravertebral block: a preliminary report of 36 cases with radiologic confirmation of catheter position. *Reg Anesth Pain Med.* 35,212–16.

Renes SH, van Geffen GJ, Snoeren MM, et al. (2011) Ipsilateral brachial plexus block and hemidiaphragmatic paresis as adverse effect of a high thoracic paravertebral block. *Reg Anesth Pain Med.* 36,198–201.

Richardson J, Lönnqvist PA. (1998) Thoracic paravertebral block. *Br J Anaesth.* 81,230–8.

Visoiu M, Yang C. (2011) Ultrasound-guided bilateral paravertebral continuous nerve blocks for a mildly coagulopathic patient undergoing exploratory laparotomy for bowel resection. *Paediatr Anaesth.* 21,459–62.

Visoiu M, Joy LN, Grudziak JS, et al. (2014) The effectiveness of ambulatory continuous peripheral nerve blocks for postoperative pain management in children and adolescents. *Paediatr Anaesth.* 24,1141–8.

Yoo SH, Lee DH, Moon DE, et al. (2012) Anatomical investigations for appropriate needle positioning for thoracic paravertebral blockade in children. *J Int Med Res.* 40,2370–80.

Chapter

18

Ultrasound-guided epidural anesthesia

Chrystelle Sola and Christophe Dadure

Clinical use

In infants and children, epidural analgesia has been proven to be a major component of the multimodal approach to perioperative pain management. Most commonly used in combination with general anesthesia, the benefits of epidural anesthesia/analgesia include a reduction of the surgical stress response, decreases in the consumption of intraoperative hypnotic agents and opioids, and the clinical impact of these reductions on post-operative ventilatory function. After surgery, the potential advantages of epidural analgesia include improved comfort with excellent pain control. This facilitates earlier extubation, improved gut function, and more rapid recovery (Walker and Yaksh, 2012; Goeller et al., 2014). Additionally, the reduction in the dose of general anesthetic agents may be desirable, particularly in infants and neonates, given the concerns regarding their potential neurotoxicity recently raised in the pediatric literature (Sinner et al., 2014). The main perioperative indications of epidural anesthesia/analgesia are major thoracic, abdominal and urologic procedures, spinal surgeries, and complex or bilateral lower limb surgeries. Outside of the operative room, the use of epidural blockade is now also well reported for chronic pain relief, such as pain associated with burns, sickle cell crisis, malignancies, or complex regional pain syndrome (Dadure et al., 2013). As with any other regional anesthesia technique, side effects may be related to placement of the needle and catheter, to the infused drugs, or to the physiologic effects of the medication. The potential list of complications of epidural anesthesia in children is the same as those in adults. However, the incidence of serious (<1:10 000) or major (<1:100 000) incidents appears rarer and less frequent than in adults. Most adverse events reported

are minor technical incidents, such as catheter-related problems (dislodgement, leakage, occlusion, or disconnection), or predictable effects, such as urinary retention and other effects associated with opioid adjuvants. Fortunately major neurologic complications are extremely rare, but infections associated with epidural catheters should always be monitored for, particularly in children at risk. Overall the infection rate is low, but prolonged use of a continuous catheter technique (>5 days) is likely to increase this risk (Sethna et al., 2010). Regarding orthopedic surgery, a recent editorial suggested that post-operative epidural analgesia does not delay the diagnosis of compartment syndrome (Johnson and Chalkiadis, 2009).

Advances in epidural analgesia are marked by the recent popularity of ultrasound-guided techniques. In the pediatric population, the use of ultrasound before and/or during an epidural block to check the anatomy provides a greater sense of safety and a high rate of success due to rapid and reliable estimation of epidural space depth, optimal determination of the needle insertion point and insertion angle (Rapp et al., 2005; Kil et al., 2007; Willschke et al., 2007; Tsui and Pillay, 2010; Tsui and Suresh, 2010).

Clinical sonoanatomy

Recent improvements in ultrasound technology have significantly enhanced our capacity to scan the vertebral structures and epidural space. These are easily identified in children due to the shallowness of the target tissue and lesser ossification of the posterior vertebral column (cartilaginous structures are sonographically transparent). This is especially true in the neonates and infants up to 6 months of age in whom direct visualization of the intrathecal space is possible. These anatomic considerations involve the use of a

---

high frequency linear probe in most cases, except in older children and adolescents where the depth of neuraxial structures may require low frequency ultrasound transducers.

Among the various sonographic views described, two main scanning planes are conventionally used and complement each other in order to obtain the relevant acoustic windows in assessing vertebro-spinal sonoanatomy (Provenzano and Narouze, 2013).

The axial scan provides a transverse view of the vertebral and intervertebral spaces. The spinal canal is bounded anteriorly by the posterior margin of vertebral body, laterally by pedicles, on which run the spinal nerves, and posteriorly by the posterior vertebra wall. The major features of the posterior vertebra wall may be easily identified: in the midline, the spinous processes appear as a hyperechoic line with a dark posterior acoustic shadow that completely hides the underlying spinal canal. Laterally on each side of the spinous process and deeper, the laminae, and in some cases articular processes of the facets joints, generate horizontal hyperechoic lines. Between the lamina and spinous process, paraspinal

muscles can be seen as two masses with different degrees of echogenicity. These are inserted deep to the transverse process and seen as a hyperechoic oblique line. At the intervertebral level, it is possible to view the contents of the vertebral canal. The characteristic image is of two hyperechoic parallel lines that are, from posterior to anterior, the ligamentum flavum and the posterior dura mater between which lies the epidural space. Deep to the dura mater, in the intrathecal space, an ultrasound scan of the spinal cord reveals a hypoechoic oval structure surrounded by a hyperechoic outline that is the pia mater. In the center of the cord, the hyperechoic dot is the paramedian sulcus. When the probe is moved in the caudal direction, the cauda equina appears as multiple, hyperechoic dots and linear structures within the thecal sac and the anechoic space is occupied by cerebrospinal fluid (Figure 18.1). The deepest hyperechoic signal reflects the posterior surface of the vertebral body. In some cases, a transverse view of the inferior spine shows normal cardiac and respiratory oscillations. Note that the skin-to-epidural space or skin-to-intrathecal space distances may be accurately

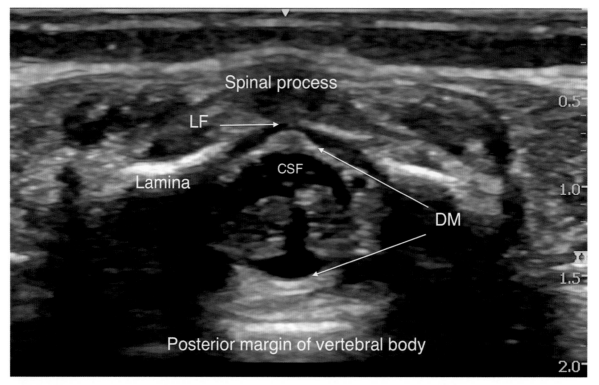

Figure 18.1 Transverse ultrasound imaging of the lumbar vertebral level L3–L4 in a 1-month-old infant. Epidural space lies between the ligamentum flavum (LF) and the posterior dura mater (DM). Note the anterior placement of the cauda equina fibers (hyperechoic dot and linear structures) within the thecal sac and the anechoic space occupied by the cerebrospinal fluid.

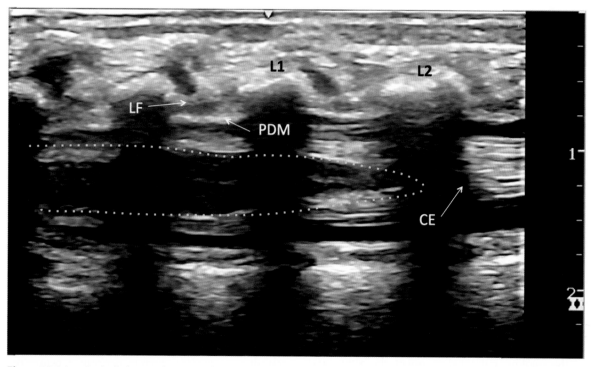

Figure 18.2 Longitudinal ultrasound imaging of the lumbar vertebral in a 1-month infant. Epidural space lies between the ligamentum flavum (LF) and the posterior dura mater (PDM). Cauda equina (CE) produces multiple horizontal hyperechoic striae. The yellow dotted line represents the conus medullaris.

assessed in this sonographic "trans-epinous" axial window.

The sagittal scan provides a wide longitudinal view of several intervertebral spaces (Figure 18.2). A paramedian approach gives the best position to visualize the neuraxis. The first osseous structure visualized appears as a "sawtooth" hyperechoic line characteristic of the complex formed by the spinous process and lamina. Superficially, the erector spinae muscles lie on the lamina. In contrast, when the transducer moves laterally, the sonographic appearance of the articular processes of the facets joint produces an unbroken hyperechoic line. Through the intermittent interlaminae acoustic windows, the spinal canal is visible – posteriorly, the ligamentum flavum and dura mater forms two highly hyperechogenic lines. The epidural space is a thin hypoechoic linear zone between these two hyperechoic lines. During the initial scanning or scout scan at the L3/4 and L4/5 interlaminar spaces, the nerve roots comprising the cauda equina lie in the anterior portion of the thecal sac and produce multiple horizontal hyperechoic striae. Cranial translation of the probe allows determination of the level of the conus medullaris (Figure 18.2). In children older than 1 year of age,

the normal position is classically established within the confines of the lower third of the body of L1 and the upper third of L2. In the neonate, the normal spinal anatomy is such that the spinal cord ends lower down the vertebral column at L3/4 and usually at the top of the body of L3 in a term infant or the bottom of the body of L3 in a preterm infant. In the sagittal view, cephalad to the conus, spinal cord is broadly hypoechoic with hyperechoic outer layer due to the reflection of the pia mater and a central line of hyperechogenicity reflecting the median sulcus.

Landmarks

In the most common situation where the child is anesthetized, the patient is placed in the lateral decubitus position with the knees drawn up to the chest and the head bent forward. Ultrasonography provides useful pre-puncture information on neuraxial structures, such as the location of the position of the conus medullaris and the dural sac and the detection of unknown structural abnormalities. Furthermore, knowledge of the ideal intervertebral level of skin puncture, on the one hand, and of the angle and depth of needle insertion, on the other hand, enhances and improves the safety of the procedure (Grau et al., 2001; Tsui and Suresh, 2010). The main objective involves identifying the target intervertebral space that correlates with the required innervation for the surgical procedure and to estimate the depth of the epidural and intrathecal spaces. Both the transverse and longitudinal views are useful for this pre-procedural evaluation.

Block performance

Ultrasound scanning of the neuraxis is more complicated than peripheral blocks and multiple views are often required to generate a complete picture of the sonoanatomy. Each view has particular benefits and limitations – a combination of scanning positions may offer the best approach.

In the longitudinal approach or scan, the paramedian window appears to provide the best access for a sonoanatomic review of the spine (Grau et al., 2001). The probe is placed parallel to the long axis of the vertebral column, just lateral to the spinous processes in the midline and tilted to orient the ultrasound beam in a medial direction toward the median sagittal plane (Figure 18.3). For the transverse scan, the transducer is rotated through 90 degrees and positioned perpendicular to the spine between 2 spinous processes to get free of the acoustic shadow (Figure 18.4).

It should be noted that ultrasound neuraxial blocks are generally using ultrasonography as "assistance," although real-time ultrasound *guidance* for epidural block techniques has also been reported in children (Rapp et al., 2005; Willschke et al., 2007). This practice is still in its infancy in clinical practice

because of the complexity of its implementation requiring frequently the need for an extra pair of hands dedicated to handling the ultrasound probe. However, direct visualization of drug spread, concomitant ventral movement of the dura mater, and the expansion of the epidural space, confirm the epidural location while the catheter insertion can be identified and visualized immediately.

According to body weight and the morphology of the child, the size of a blunt tip "Tuohy" type needle is carefully determined (Table 18.1): for neonates, a 20-gauge 50 mm needle combined with a 24-gauge catheter is advocated. An intermediate 19-gauge needle with 24-gauge catheter is also suitable for an infant until 6 months of age. For older children, an 18-gauge needle and 20-gauge catheter is commonly used.

In the most cases, a linear probe with a 25–38 mm probe surface length and an ultrasound frequency from 8 to 18 MHz provides accurate imaging of anatomic structures. In older children and adolescents, the depth of neuraxial structures may require the use of low frequency ultrasound and curved array transducers. Preview imaging performed before the epidural procedure is an excellent tool to identify neuraxial structures in both infants and children. In addition, epidural catheter placement under a real-time ultrasound guidance technique has shown a high rate of success in neonatal and infant populations (Rapp et al., 2005; Willschke et al., 2007) and could become the standard of practice in the future.

The midline needle approach with a paramedian longitudinal scan allows an in-plane needle insertion, offering a better acoustic window and the most useful visualization of neuraxial structures (Figure 18.3).

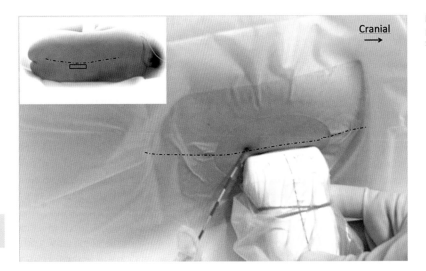

Figure 18.3 Patient position with probe placement for paramedian longitudinal scan and in-plane Tuohy needle insertion.

Table 18.1 Needle size, local anesthetic, and adjuvant doses for epidural continuous anesthesia in children

Age (months)		<1	1–6	>6
Tuohy needle		20-G 50 mm	19 / 20-G 50 mm	18-G 50 / 80 mm
Drug Induction dose	Concentration	Levobupivacaine 0.125% Ropivacaine 0.1%	Levobupivacaine 0.125%-0.25% Ropivacaine 0.1%-0.2%	Levobupivacaine 0.25% Ropivacaine 0.2%
	Volume	0.5-0.7 ml/kg (max 1.6 mg/kg)	05–0.7 ml/kg (max 1.8 mg/kg)	0.5-0.7 ml/kg (max 2 mg/kg or 15 ml)
	Adjuvant (µg / ml LA)	-	Clonidine 0.5–1 µg/ml Sufentanil 0.1–0.5 µg/ml Fentanyl 0.5–1 µg/ml	Clonidine 0.5-1 µg/ml Sufentanil 0.1-0.5 µg/ml Fentanyl 0.5-1 µg/ml
Drug Infusion dose	Concentration	Levobupivacaine 0.125% Ropivacaine 0.1%	Levobupivacaine 0.125% Ropivacaine 0.1%	Levobupivacaine 0.25% Ropivacaine 0.2%
	Maintenance Adjuvant (µg/ml LA)	0.2 ml/kg/h -	0.2 ml/kg/h Clonidine 0.5–1µg/ml Sufentanil 0.1–0.2 µg/ml Fentanyl 0.5–1 µg/ml	0.2 ml/kg/h Clonidine 0.5-1µg/ml Sufentanil 0.1-0.2 µg/ml Fentanyl 0.5-1 µg/ml
PCEA NCEA		-	-	Basal: 0.08-0.1 ml/kg/ h Bolus: 0.1 ml/kg/h Refractory period: 20-30mn Max/h: 0.2 ml/kg/h

G, gauge; LA, local anesthetic; PCEA, patient-controlled epidural analgesia; NCEA, nurse-controlled epidural analgesia.

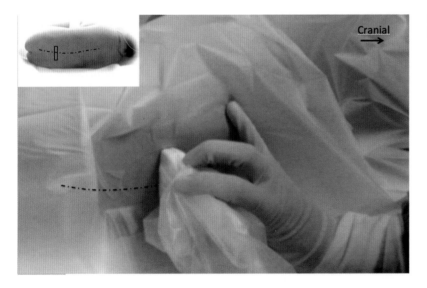

Cranial →

Figure 18.4 Patient position with probe placement for transverse view.

The correct position of the needle into the epidural space is clearly identified by direct vision of the saline solution spread associated with anterior displacement of the posterior dura mater and widening of the epidural space. Once the appropriate location of the needle tip is confirmed, the catheter is inserted to a maximum of 2–3 cm into the epidural space to avoid kinking or knotting of the catheter. In some children, generally infants less than 6 months of age, direct tracking of catheter placement is possible but this is not consistent. However, using multiple imaging planes and based on indirect markers such as tissue movement and by fluid injection, the catheter tip position can be appreciated even in older children. A recent study demonstrated that real-time ultrasound guidance resulted in shorter procedure times and less unwanted bone contact

129

during the procedure while providing a high degree of safety throughout (Perlas, 2010).

Post-operative care

The primary objective of an epidural catheter is to provide effective intraoperative site specific anesthesia and optimal post-operative analgesia. Established protocols of care, carried out in a suitable ward or unit and with the continuous vigilance of trained staff, are prerequisites for setting up a continuous epidural infusion service. To prevent potential local and systemic toxicity of the local anesthetic (LA), especially in neonates and infants where the risk of drug accumulation after a continuous infusion is increased, the choice of the concentration and the volume of the solution should be carefully evaluated (Table 18.1). Newer LA agents (ropivacaine and levobupivacaine) provide at low concentration, a differential blocking effect on nerve fibers, less intense motor blockade consequently, and similar satisfactory analgesia compared to bupivacaine. A continuous infusion of a low LA concentration solution at 0.2 mg/kg/h in infants and 0.4 mg/kg/h in older children has been shown to be an effective and safe dosage. Effective pain relief can be obtained in some children by using an epidural patient controlled analgesia with subsequent lower dose requirements than a continuous epidural infusion (Antok et al., 2003). Adjuvant drugs are commonly used to improve the duration and quality of the LA blockade. Opioids such as fentanyl, morphine, and sufentanil are often used but require monitoring of respiratory function. Alpha-2 agonists such as clonidine can often play a key role in improving post-operative analgesia without concerns regarding respiratory compromise.

Despite the increasing use of ultrasound in neuraxial techniques, there is currently insufficient data to demonstrate improvements in the outcome of ultrasound assisted or guided neuraxial blocks in children (Rubin et al., 2009). Nevertheless, the use of non-invasive ultrasound imaging techniques has brought about a revolutionary advance in neuraxial anesthesia and analgesia for pediatric patients.

Suggested reading

Antok E, Bordet F., Duflo, F., et al. (2003) Patient-controlled epidural analgesia versus continuous epidural infusion with ropivacaine for postoperative analgesia in children. *Anesth Analg.* 97,1608–11.

Dadure C, Marec P, Veyckmans F, Beloeil H. (2013) Chronic pain and regional anesthesia in children. *Arch Pediatr.* 20,1149–57.

Goeller JK, Bhalla T, Tobias JD. (2014) Combined use of neuraxial and general anesthesia during major abdominal procedures in neonates and infants. *Paediatr Anaesth.* 24,553–60.

Grau T, Leipold RW, Conradi R, Martin E. (2001) Ultrasound control for presumed difficult epidural puncture. *Acta Anaesthesiol Scand.* 45,766–71.

Johnson DJ, Chalkiadis GA. (2009) Does epidural analgesia delay the diagnosis of lower limb compartment syndrome in children? *Paediatr Anaesth.* 19,83–91.

Kil HK, Cho JE, Kim WO, et al. (2007) Prepuncture ultrasound-measured distance: an accurate reflection of epidural depth in infants and small children. *Reg Anesth Pain Med.* 32,102–6.

Perlas A. (2010) Evidence for the use of ultrasound in neuraxial blocks. *Reg Anesth Pain Med.* 35,S43–6.

Provenzano DA, Narouze S. (2013) Sonographically guided lumbar spine procedures. *J Ultrasound Med.* 32,1109–16.

Rapp HJ, Folger A, Grau T. (2005) Ultrasound-guided epidural catheter insertion in children. *Anesth Analg.* 101,333–9.

Rubin K, Sullivan D, Sadhasivam S. (2009) Are peripheral and neuraxial blocks with ultrasound guidance more effective and safe in children? *Paediatr Anaesth.* 19,92–6.

Sethna NF, Clendenin D, Athiraman U, et al. (2010) Incidence of epidural catheter-associated infections after continuous epidural analgesia in children. *Anesthesiology.* 113,224–32.

Sinner B, Becke K, Engelhard K. (2014) General anaesthetics and the developing brain: an overview. *Anaesthesia.* 69,1009–22.

Tsui BC, Pillay JJ. (2010) Evidence-based medicine: assessment of ultrasound imaging for regional anesthesia in infants, children, and adolescents. *Reg Anesth Pain Med.* 35,S47–54.

Tsui BC, Suresh S. (2010) Ultrasound imaging for regional anesthesia in infants, children, and adolescents: a review of current literature and its application in the practice of neuraxial blocks. *Anesthesiology.* 112,719–28.

Walker SM, Yaksh TL. (2012) Neuraxial analgesia in neonates and infants: a review of clinical and preclinical strategies for the development of safety and efficacy data. *Anesth Analg.* 115,638–62.

Willschke H, Bosenberg A, Marhofer P, et al. (2007) Epidural catheter placement in neonates: sonoanatomy and feasibility of ultrasonographic guidance in term and preterm neonates. *Reg Anesth Pain Med.* 32,34–40.

Chapter

19

Ultrasound for spinal anesthesia

Karthikeyan Kallidaikurichi Srinivasan and Peter Lee

Clinical use

The use of ultrasound to aid pediatric spinal anesthesia is a relatively recent advancement. Ultrasound imaging of the neuraxis in children (especially in infants <6 months of age) is a simpler task than in adults, as a result of a largely cartilaginous posterior vertebral column. It is still considered an advanced imaging technique due to the limited ultrasound window. Absence of the ossification associated with ageing greatly increases penetration by the ultrasound beam, thereby producing a clearer image of neuraxial structures. Structures not normally seen in scans of the adult neuraxis (spinal cord, conus medullaris, cauda equina, vertebral body) and even the spread of local anesthetic (LA) in the epidural space may be visualized in infants (Chawathe et al., 2003). Although ultrasound images of neuraxial structures are more limited with increasing age due to ossification of posterior elements, it can still be useful in identifying structures of interest in older children (Marhofer et al., 2005).

Spinal anesthesia in pediatrics is usually done in the patient population at risk of post-operative apnea (e.g. ex-preterm infants, muscular dystrophy) and in a patient population predisposed to chronic lung disease (e.g. bronchopulmonary dysplasia) to minimize airway manipulation. It is suitable as a sole anesthetic agent for infraumbilical surgeries (e.g. inguinal hernia repair, urologic surgeries, lower limb orthopedic procedures). In addition to a reduction in the incidence of post-operative apnea, hypoxia, and bradycardia, spinal anesthesia also contributes to a blunting of the neuroendocrine response.

The procedure does have its own limitations with a number of differences from adult practice. The duration of action is short, lasting for 60–90 minutes. Failure rates have been reported to be as high as 28%

with a higher incidence of bloody tap (8–19%). The incidence of post-dural puncture headache (8–25%) also tends to be higher than in adult population. In addition to routine contraindications to neuraxial procedures (allergy to LA, active local or systemic infection, and coagulopathy), anatomic contraindications, such as occult spinal dysraphism and meningomyelocoele, are also relevant in this age group. Proceeding in cases with intracerebral hemorrhage and hydrocephalus should be based on a risk–benefit analysis for each patient.

Neuraxial ultrasound yields numerous details of spinal anatomy relevant to the administration of spinal anesthesia. The spinal cord terminates at the L3–L4 vertebral body in the newborn and gradually ascends to end between the L1 and L2 vertebral bodies towards the end of the first year of life. Therefore, in pediatric patients, spinal anesthesia should be performed at or below the L4–L5 vertebrae to minimize the risk of trauma to the spinal cord. Ultrasound has been used successfully to identify interspinous levels in a pediatric population (Hayes et al., 2014).

Ultrasound can be used to estimate the distance from the skin to the ligamentum flavum. In 180 children aged between 2 and 84 months, ultrasound-based estimation of the depth of the ligamentum flavum had a high correlation for both longitudinal and transverse views (Kil et al., 2007). Estimation of that depth in older children was also shown to be feasible in a study of 137 children aged between 7 and 12 years (Ozer et al., 2005). In smaller infants, estimation of the depth of the spinal canal is particularly important as needle advancement beyond the spinal canal can lead to trauma to the posterior vertebral body and associated venous plexus (Arthurs et al., 2008).

Ultrasound-Guided Regional Anesthesia in Children, ed. Mannion et al. Published by Cambridge University Press.
© Cambridge University Press 2015.

Ultrasound may also be useful in determining the best angle of insertion for the spinal needle and the identification of difficult or abnormal anatomy. In a study of 36 children aged 0–12 years, ultrasound visualization of the spinous processes aided calculation of needle insertion angle into the subarachnoid space (Bruccoleri and Chen, 2011). Ultrasound may be used to identify anatomic anomalies (low-lying cord, tethered cord syndrome, caudal regression syndrome) and, therefore, alert the anesthesiologist to avoid spinal anesthesia in this group of children. Spinal ultrasound is equivalent to spinal magnetic resonance imaging (MRI) in identifying these conditions (Dick and de Bruyn, 2003).

Ultrasound-guided techniques have been successfully used in children with a high body mass index (Kawaguchi et al., 2007), previous spinal surgery, scoliosis, and with a history of prior difficult dural puncture (Warhadpande et al., 2013).

There are a few limitations of ultrasound-guided spinal anesthesia in children:

1. Much of the current evidence is based on the use of ultrasound in the performance of lumbar puncture or depth estimation for epidural cannulation. There is a lack of data comparing success rates between conventional and ultrasound-guided techniques for spinal anesthesia in children.

2. Due to the uncooperative nature of the pediatric population for invasive procedures, the time available to perform the procedure safely may be limited. With experience, the additional time required for scanning should be negligible.

3. Neuraxial ultrasound, a relatively novel skill for many anesthesiologists, has a steep learning curve.

4. The safety of ultrasound gel for neuraxial block is still unclear (Belavy et al., 2013; Hampl et al., 2014)

Although the current limited available evidence does not support the *routine* use of ultrasound for pediatric spinal anesthesia, it has a definite role in specific population groups where the administration of spinal anesthesia can be difficult or in the presence of suspected anatomic abnormality.

Clinical sonoanatomy

The sonoanatomy of the neuraxis depends on the orientation of probe:

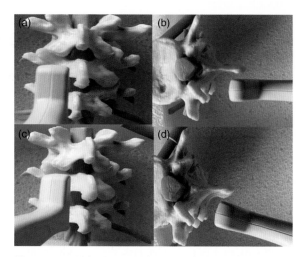

Figure 19.1 Probe position. (a,b) Paramedian sagittal (PS) view probe position – view from behind and above. (c,d) Paramedian sagittal oblique (PSO) view probe position – view from behind and above.

a. Paramedian sagittal (PS) view (Figure 19.1a,b) – the probe is placed in a sagittal plane lateral and parallel to midline.

b. Paramedian sagittal oblique (PSO) view (Figure 19.1c,d) – the probe is positioned as for PS view but with a slight tilt of the probe towards the midline.

c. Transverse median (TM) view – the probe is positioned in a transverse plane.

Sagittal views

The scanning starts with the PS view with the probe positioned over the sacrum. In infants the sacral segments are not fused and so the first sacral segment is identified by its dorsal tilt (Dick and de Bruyn, 2003). The L5–S1 junction is the point between the obliquely oriented first sacral vertebra and the horizontally oriented fifth lumbar vertebra (Figure 19.2). Close attention to this is important as estimation of interspinous space is dependent on this (in older children the sacrum may be identified as a continuous convex hyperechoic line).

Once the first sacral vertebra is identified then the probe is moved cephalad in the same orientation to identify the L5 and L4 laminae. Alternatively, the vertebral level may be determined by identifying the twelfth thoracic vertebra based on its articulation with the last rib, and thereafter moving the probe in a caudal direction. The first method tends to be more reliable (Deeg et al., 2007).

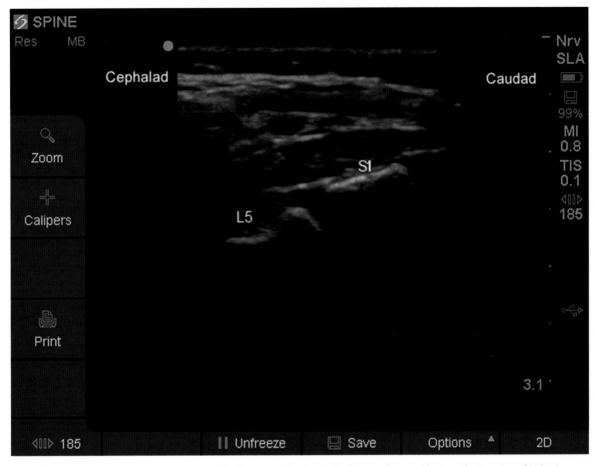

Figure 19.2 L5–S1 interlaminar view (3-month-old infant). Note the dorsal tilt of S1 vertebrae and horizontal orientation of L5 lamina.

A slight angulation of the probe to point towards the midline improves the view of neuraxial structures through the interlaminar window. This is the paramedian sagittal oblique (PSO) view.

The structures typically seen in PSO view are (Figures 19.3 and 19.4):

1. Lamina
2. Posterior complex (PC) consisting of ligamentum flavum and posterior dura mater (in infants the dura mater is better visualized than ligamentum flavum).
3. Hypoechoic spinal canal
4. Filum terminale along with cauda equina (visualized better in infants where it is seen as closely related parallel lines extending from conus).
5. Anterior complex (AC) consisting of the anterior dura mater, posterior longitudinal ligament, and posterior surface of the vertebral body.

6. In infants younger than 6 months of age, conus medullaris and spinal cord (visualized as a hypoechoic cylindrical structure with central echogenic complex) can be seen in the spinal canal between the hyper-echoic anterior and posterior dura mater.

Probe marking from PSO view

Once the appropriate interlaminar space (L4–L5 or L5–S1) is identified for spinal anesthesia, the probe positions are marked. With the interlaminar space of interest in the middle of the ultrasound screen, the midpoint of the long border of the probe is marked on either side of the probe using a skin marker. As the ultrasound beam emanates from the middle of the probe, the midpoint between the two markings should correspond to the selected interspace.

133

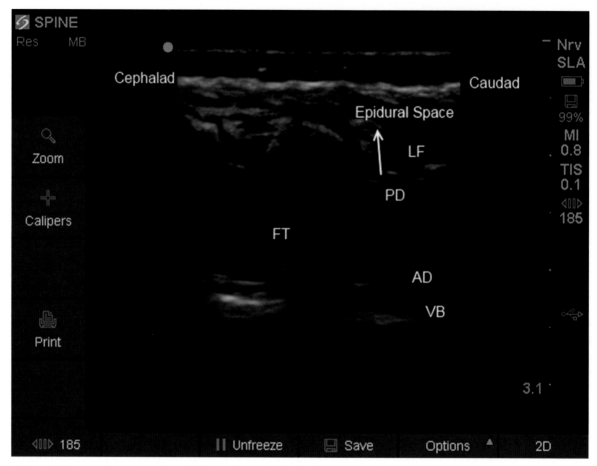

Figure 19.3 Paramedian sagittal oblique (PSO) view (3-month-old infant). AD, anterior dura mater; FT, filum terminale; LF, ligamentum flavum; PD, posterior dura mater; VB, vertebral body.

Transverse median view

Following the skin marking in the PSO view, the probe is turned 90 degrees to obtain a transverse median (TM) view at the same level.

Structures seen when probe is placed directly over the spinous process include (Figure 19.5):

1. A superficial hyperechoic line of the spinous process.
2. Hyperechoic lamina on either side of the spinous process.

The probe is moved just below or above the spinous process, to lessen the acoustic impedance of interspinous ligaments compared to spinous processes. This window provides a clearer image of neuraxial structures which include (Figure 19.6):

1. Two hyperechoic lines are seen in the midline – this denotes PC and AC.

2. Two hyperechoic lines on either side of the midline – this represents the transverse process on either side (note at this level, as the probe is below the spinous process and lamina, the hyperechoic structures seen are the transverse process).
3. In infants – cauda equina and filum terminale can be seen as hyperechoic structures within spinal canal with spinal cord itself seen as a tubular hypoechoic structure with a hyperechoic central complex.

Probe marking for TM view

On obtaining the best view with the image positioned in the middle of the ultrasound screen, the midpoint of the sides of the probe and midpoint of the short ends of the probe are marked. The intersection of the two lines will provide the needle insertion point.

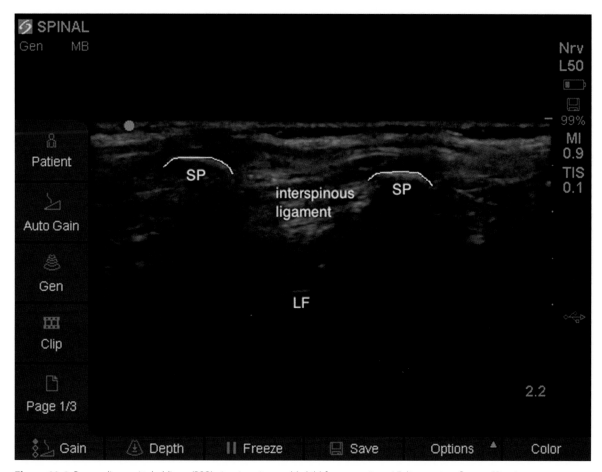

Figure 19.4 Paramedian sagittal oblique (PSO) view in a 4-year-old child for comparison. LF, ligamentum flavum; SP, spinous process.

Block performance

In small children and infants, linear probes with a high frequency (7–13 MHz) are preferred to curvilinear (curved array) probes (Marhofer et al., 2005). A smaller probe (e.g. "hockey-stick" probes) may allow more accurate placement of skin markings. For older children, in whom the depth of the intrathecal space is greater than 4 cm, a curvilinear probe may be more suitable.

Although real-time ultrasound guidance for epidural catheter insertions in children has been previously described (Rapp et al., 2005; Willschke et al., 2006), a similar technique has not been studied for the administration of spinal anesthesia in children. In children, administering subarachnoid block using real-time ultrasound guidance might be possible; however, this area needs further research. The following description is for pre-procedural ultrasound with skin marking followed by performance of spinal anesthesia. The term "ultrasound assisted" is more appropriate than "ultrasound guidance."

Ultrasound scanning can be performed with the child in the lateral decubitus or lateral position (with or without a 45-degree head-up tilt) or in the sitting position. Lateral decubitus position with 45-degree head-up tilt resulted in significantly higher incidence of successful dural puncture compared to lateral decubitus position alone (Apiliogullari et al., 2008) (Figure 19.7). In all three positions the assistant holding the child should ensure that the neck is maintained in a neutral position as flexion of the neck may lead to desaturation, bradycardia, and reduction in PaO_2 (Spahr et al.,1981; Weisman et al.,1983; Fiser et al., 1993). Neck flexion does not improve the visibility but increases associated morbidity (Abo et al., 2010).

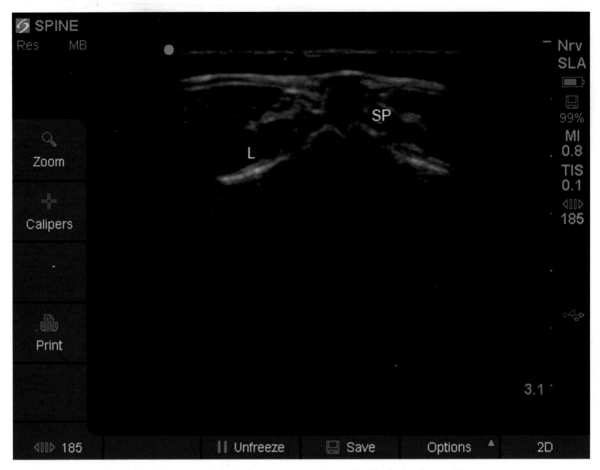

Figure 19.5 Transverse median (TM) view at the level of spinous process (3-month-old infant). L, lamina; SP, spinous process.

There is no difference in the dimensions of the lumbar subarachnoid space when measured by ultrasound between the three positions (Lo et al., 2013). Use of the lateral flexed position results in an increase in the interspinous distance compared to a neutral position in children under 1 month of age (Cadigan et al., 2011). A sitting position with flexed hips also significantly increases the interspinous distance in children younger than 12 years (Abo et al., 2010).

Initial placement of the probe should be in PSO orientation in the sacrococcygeal area. Palpation of posterior superior iliac crest and sacral cornua should help to identify this. The intercristal line (Tuffier's line) may correspond to L4–L5 or L3–L4 interspinous space but should be confirmed by ultrasound. Once the L4–L5 or L5–S1 interlaminar space is identified, skin markings are made as detailed earlier. The depth of the subarachnoid space from the skin (measured as

the distance between the skin and the posterior complex) is noted. The probe is rotated 90 degrees to obtain the TM view at that same level. Once satisfactory images of the PC and AC are obtained, the image is positioned in the middle of the ultrasound screen, ensuring that the transverse processes are symmetrical. Cephalo-caudal angulation of the probe is performed to optimize the image of the posterior and anterior complex. In addition the mediolateral angle is adjusted to obtain a symmetrical view of transverse process on either side. Both of these angles should be recalled by the operator to inform needle trajectory. The depth of the subarachnoid space is also estimated. Finally the skin is marked around the probe as detailed above to identify the optimal needle insertion point.

On successful entry to the subarachnoid space, the calculated dose of LA is injected slowly (Table 19.1).

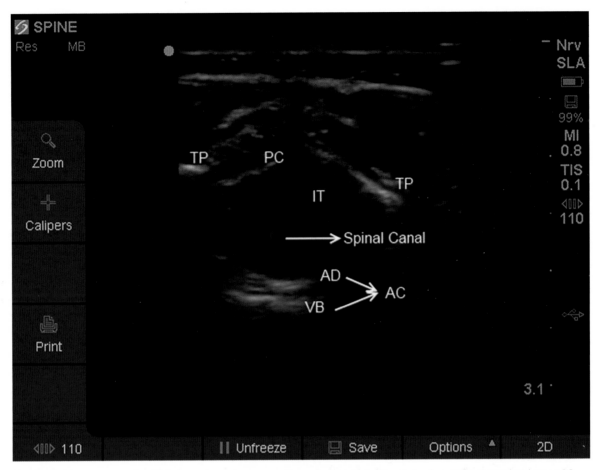

Figure 19.6 Transverse median (TM) view at interspinous space (3-month-old infant). AD, anterior dura mater; IT, intrathecal space; PC, posterior complex; TP, transverse process; VB, vertebral body. Note the spinal canal is seen as hyperechoic dot surrounded by hypoechoic spinal cord.

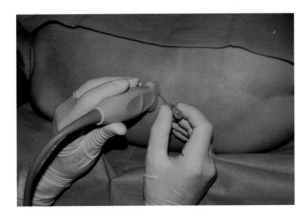

Figure 19.7 Patient position with slight neck extension. Transverse probe position.

In infants reliable assessment of block height can be difficult. The onset of motor block of the lower extremities can be seen early. Paralysis of the abdominal muscles can be seen when the child is coughing or crying. Tetanic stimulation by a peripheral nerve stimulator may also aid the assessment of block height (Rowney and Doyle, 1998).In older children, the loss of cold sensation can be used to estimate block height.

Post-operative care

As the duration of action is usually limited to less than 90 minutes, prolonged duration of action should be viewed suspiciously. Close monitoring of neurologic status is needed in most cases to avoid any delay in the recognition of serious complications. In high-risk

137

Table 19.1 Drug doses for spinal anesthesia

Drug	Up to 6 months	6 months to 14 years	Duration of action
0.5% Bupivacaine (hyper or isobaric)	0.5–0.6 mg/kg (0.10–0.12 ml/kg)	0.2–0.3 mg/kg (0.04–0.05 ml/kg)	90–120 min
0.5% Levobupivacaine	1 mg/kg (0.2 ml/kg)	0.3 mg/kg (0.05 ml/kg)	90–120 min
0.5% Tetracaine	0.5–0.6 mg/kg (0.1–0.12 ml/kg)	0.2–0.3 mg/kg (0.04–0.05 ml/kg)	60–240 min

groups, apnea monitoring is advised even when the procedure is performed under spinal anesthesia.

Clinical tips

- The ultrasound probe should be thoroughly cleaned prior to the start of sterile procedure.
- Laminae are cartilaginous in young children and so the paramedian approach should be avoided.
- The dead space of the spinal needle (0.02–0.04 ml) should be included in volume calculation.
- Inject the intrathecal LA slowly (20 s).
- Positioning after spinal anesthetic – do not lift the baby for placement of the diathermy pad.
- During surgery – pacifier/sedation/no sedation may be required depending on the age of the child.
- Note the shorter duration of action as a result of the increased volume of cerebrospinal fluid in the intrathecal space and the increased blood flow.

Suggested reading

Abo A, Chen L, Johnston P, Santucci K. (2010) Positioning for lumbar puncture in children evaluated by bedside ultrasound. *Pediatrics.* 125(5),1149–53.

Apiliogullari S, Duman A, Gok F, Ogun, CO, Akillioglu I. (2008) The effects of 45 degree head up tilt on the lumbar puncture success rate in children undergoing spinal anesthesia. *Paediatr Anaesth.* 18(12),1178–82.

Arthurs OJ, Murray M, Zubier M, Tooley J, Kelsall W. (2008) Ultrasonographic determination of neonatal spinal canal depth. *Arch Dis Child Fetal Neonatal Ed.* 93(6),451–4.

Belavy D, Sunn N, Lau Q, Robertson T. (2013) Absence of neurotoxicity with perineural injection of ultrasound gels: assessment using an animal model. *BMC Anesthesiol.* 13(1),18.

Bruccoleri RE, Chen L. (2011) Needle-entry angle for lumbar puncture in children as determined by using ultrasonography. *Pediatrics.* 127(4),921–6.

Cadigan BA, Cydulka RK, Werner SL, Jones RA. (2011) Evaluating infant positioning for lumbar puncture using sonographic measurements. *Acad Emerg Med.* 18(2),215–18.

Chawathe MS, Jones RM, Gildersleve CD, et al. (2003) Detection of epidural catheters with ultrasound in children. *Paediatr Anaesth.* 13(8),681–4.

Deeg KH, Lode HM, Gassner I. (2007). Spinal sonography in newborns and infants–Part I: method, normal anatomy and indications. *Ultraschall Med.* 28(5),507–17.

Dick EA, de Bruyn R. (2003) Ultrasound of the spinal cord in children: its role. *Eur Radiol.* 13(3),552–62.

Fiser DH, Gober GA, Smith CE, et al. (1993) Prevention of hypoxemia during lumbar puncture in infancy with preoxygenation. *Pediatr Emerg Care.* 9(2),81–3.

Hampl K, Steinfeldt T, Wulf H. (2014) Spinal anesthesia revisited: toxicity of new and old drugs and compounds. *Curr Opin Anaesthesiol.* 27(5),549–55.

Hayes J, Borges B, Armstrong D, Srinivasan I. (2014) Accuracy of manual palpation vs. ultrasound for identifying the L3–L4 intervertebral space level in children. *Paediatr Anaesth.* 24(5),510–15.

Kawaguchi R, Yamauch M, Sugino S, et al. (2007) [Two cases of epidural anesthesia using ultrasound imaging]. *Masui.* 56(6),702–5.

Kil HK, Cho JE, Kim WO, et al. (2007) Prepuncture ultrasound-measured distance: an accurate reflection of epidural depth in infants and small children. *Reg Anesth Pain Med.* 32(2),102–6.

Lo, MD, Parisi MT, Brown JC, Klein EJ. (2013) Sitting or tilt position for infant lumbar puncture does not increase ultrasound measurements of lumbar subarachnoid space width. *Pediatr Emerg Care.* 29(5),588–91.

Marhofer P, Bosenberg A, Sitzwohl C, et al. (2005) Pilot study of neuraxial imaging by ultrasound in infants and children. *Paediatr Anaesth.* 15(8),671–6.

Ozer Y, Ozer T, Altunkaya H, Savranlar A. (2005) The posterior lumbar dural depth: an ultrasonographic study in children. *Agri.* 17(3),53–7.

Rapp HJ, Folger A, Grau T. (2005) Ultrasound-guided epidural catheter insertion in children. *Anesth Analg.* 101(2),333–9.

Rowney DA, Doyle E. (1998) Epidural and subarachnoid blockade in children. *Anaesthesia.* 53(10), 980–1001.

Spahr RC, MacDonald HM, Mueller-Heubach E. (1981) Knee–chest position and neonatal oxygenation and blood pressure. *Am J Dis Child.* 135(1),79–80.

Warhadpande S, Martin D, Bhalla T, et al. (2013) Use of ultrasound to facilitate difficult lumbar puncture in the pediatric oncology population. *Int J Clin Exp Med.* 6(2),149–52.

Weisman LE, Merenstein GB, Steenbarger JR. (1983) The effect of lumbar puncture position in sick neonates. *Am J Dis Child.* 137(11),1077–9.

Willschke H, Marhofer P, Bosenberg A, et al. (2006) Epidural catheter placement in children: comparing a novel approach using ultrasound guidance and a standard loss-of-resistance technique. *Br J Anaesth.* 97(2),200–7.

Ultrasound-guided caudal block

Anca Grigoras and Jawad Mustafa

Clinical use

Caudal epidural blockade is the most frequently used regional anesthesia technique in pediatric patients. Caudal block in children provides intra- and postoperative pain control in surgical procedures below the umbilicus (perineal, genitourinary, ilioinguinal, lower extremity surgery), and it is almost always performed under general anesthesia. The technique can occasionally be used as the sole anesthetic in high-risk patients (newborn and premature infants, neuromuscular disease, malignant hyperthermia susceptibility) in order to reduce the risks associated with general anesthesia. Caudal analgesia is produced by injection of local anesthetic (LA) into the caudal canal through the sacral hiatus. The success rate depends upon accurate identification of the hiatus and an adequate needle insertion angle.

The incidence of serious complications that can result in patient harm or sequelae is very low, particularly with single shot caudal blocks. The most common adverse event associated with caudal block in children is the inability to place the block or block failure followed by urinary retention (Polaner et al., 2012).

In children, the size and position of the spinal cord is different from adults: at birth the cord ends at L3/L4 and the dura mater at S3. That may increase the risk of spine injury during advancement of the caudal needle. The distance between dural sac and hiatus varies, but it is less than 10 mm in newborns. As the child grows, the cord and the dural sac rise to reach their adult level L1/L2 and S2, respectively, by the end of the first year of life. In newborns and infants, the sacral bone is composed mostly of cartilage and soft bony tissue that increases the risk of bone penetration and rectal puncture.

Ultrasonography allows for easy identification of sacral anatomy (specifically the relation of the sacral hiatus to the dural sac and the search of occult spinal dysraphism) before attempting the block. This is particularly important in children with an anatomy that is difficult to define by palpation alone. By using ultrasound, the anesthetist can visualize the cranial spread of LA in the caudal–epidural space, or the placement of an epidural catheter. Ultrasound guidance offers a reliable caudal block for pediatric patients with the advantages of easier performance and fewer complications compared with traditional sacral canal injection (Wang et al., 2013).

Ultrasound assessment of LA spread after caudal block shows that cranial spread is dependent on the volume injected into the caudal space. However, the dermatomal difference in cranial spread in the volume range 0.7–1.3 ml/kg is only minor and difficult to predict, and unlikely to be clinically significant (Brenner et al., 2011).

Ultrasound imaging is a reliable indicator of correct needle position for caudal block. The observation of dural displacement secondary to the saline test bolus, using the in-plane approach, was reported in 93.6% of patients (Roberts et al., 2005). Ultrasonographic assessment suggests that the optimal angle of needle insertion during caudal epidural block in children is about 20 degrees to the skin surface. With this angle, the chance of performing a successful caudal injection can be increased with minimal risk of intraosseous insertion (Park et al., 2006).

Increased ossification of the spine in older children can diminish the quality of the ultrasound view when performing the block or positioning the caudally inserted epidural catheters (Roberts and Galvez, 2005).

Clinical sonoanatomy

The caudal space can be visualized in two views, transverse and longitudinal.

Ultrasound-Guided Regional Anesthesia in Children, ed. Mannion et al. Published by Cambridge University Press.
© Cambridge University Press 2015.

Transverse scan

The scan shows two hyperechoic sacral cornua and dark acoustic shadows posterior to each of them. The hyperechoic fibrous structure intervening between them, deep to the skin and subcutaneous tissue, is the sacrococcygeal membrane or ligament. The two sacral cornua and the posterior surface of the sacrum produce an ultrasound image described as the "frog-eye sign" because of its resemblance to the eyes of a frog. Posterior to the sacrococcygeal membrane is the base of the sacrum (Figure 20.1).

Longitudinal scan

The sagital sonogram of the sacrum shows the sacro-coccygeal ligament, the base of the sacrum, and the sacral hiatus. In neonates and young infants the tapered end of the dural sac with cerebrospinal fluid (CSF), the cauda equine, and the anterior and posterior epidural space filled with fat may be visualized in the sacral canal. The dura mater is hyperechoic and forms the anterior and posterior border of the subarachnoid space (Figure 20.2).

Landmarks

The patient is usually in the left lateral position with the knees drawn up to the chest. Flexing helps to palpate the sacral cornua better and brings the end of the dural sac cranially. Successful performance of a caudal epidural starts with the accurate identification of the sacral hiatus. The sacral hiatus lies at the third point of an equilateral triangle formed with the two posterior superior iliac spines (look for the dimples in the skin). The cornua are palpable on either side of the hiatus. Two cornua are easily palpable in infants and children, and the sacrococcygeal membrane is sometimes visible through the skin because of the absence of the sacral fat pad, which usually develops at puberty.

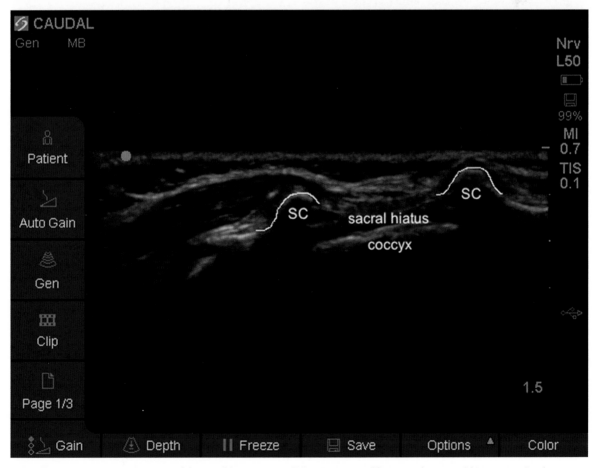

Figure 20.1 Transverse sonoanatomy of the sacral (sacrum cornu (SC), sacrococcygeal ligament above sacral hiatus, coccyx) – the "frog eye sign."

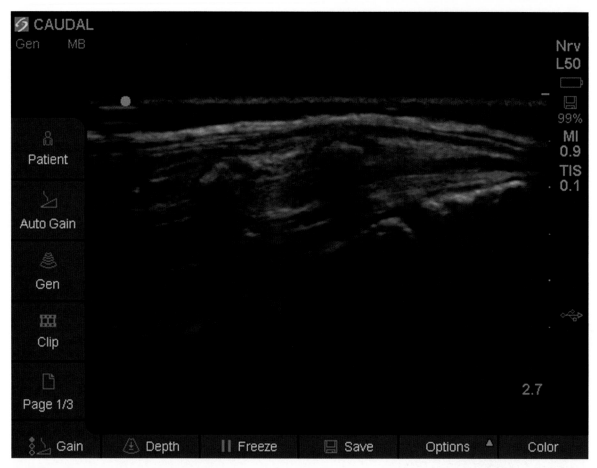

Figure 20.2 Sagittal sonoanatomy of the sacrum.

The probe is positioned directly over the sacral cornua in the transverse plane to obtain a transverse view of the sacral hiatus (Figure 20.3). The transducer can be rotated in the sagittal plane and placed between the two cornua to obtain a longitudinal view of the caudal space (Figure 20.4). When anatomic landmarks are difficult to identify, the placement of the probe at the level of coccyx with subsequent scanning toward the sacral canal will help clinician to localize relevant structures.

Block performance

The child is placed in the lateral position and the landmarks for caudal puncture are identified (Figure 20.3).

Ultrasound imaging is performed using a high frequency linear array probe. The linear ultrasound probes with a 38-mm active surface area (or probes with 25-mm active surface area in smaller children), with high frequencies in the range 8–14 MHz, allow a good compromise between excellent resolution for superficial structures and good penetration depths. Caudal needles (22-gauge/35 mm or 20-gauge/50 mm) with a dull Crawford type bevel and precision-ground stylets in order to minimize tissue coring are recommended. Depth and gain settings are adjusted for optimal image quality.

The ultrasound probe covered with a sterile sheath is placed between the sacral cornua in sagittal plane and the needle is advanced under real-time guidance into the sacral canal through the sacrococcygeal ligament. With in-plane technique the entire length of the needle can be visualized, including the tip (Figure 20.5). The needle is advanced at an angle of approximately 20 degrees, so that it is parallel to the posterior surface of the sacrum and the risk of insertion into deeper structures is low. Once a "pop" is felt and/or the needle is visualized on the sonogram, the correct position of the needle in the caudal epidural space has to be confirmed. This is done by injecting a test bolus of saline (0.1–0.2 ml/kg) and observing in

real-time the anterior displacement of posterior dura. The use of saline prevents wastage of LA with inadequate needle positioning, and if injected intravascularly or intrathecally does not put the patient at risk. Absence of dura displacement could be associated with intrathecal or intravascular positioning of the needle. The needle should be withdrawn and repositioned. After confirming the correct placement of the needle, the calculated dose of LA (Table 20.1) is injected in aliquots. The cephalad spread of the LA within the epidural space can be visualized by the use of color Doppler.

With the out-of-plane approach, the sacral hiatus is firstly scanned at the sacral cornua in a transverse plane (Figure 20.1). With the ultrasound image of hiatus in the middle of ultrasound screen, the puncture site is positioned caudad adjacent to the midpoint of the transducer. Once a "pop" is felt and/or the needle is visualized in the hiatus a test

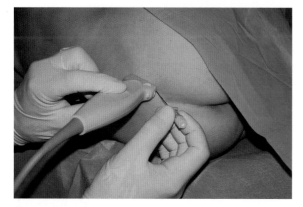

Figure 20.3 Patient position, probe placement, and in-plane needle technique.

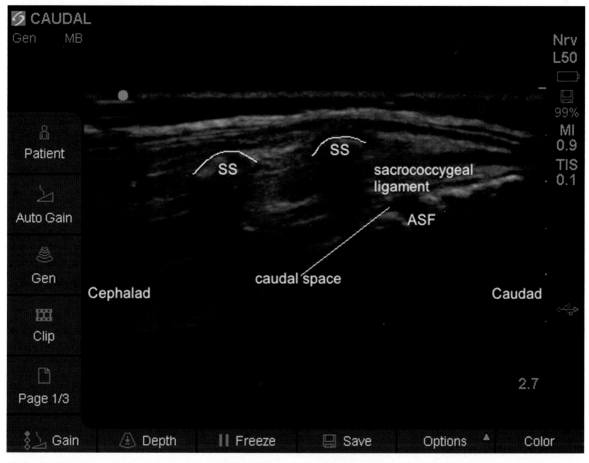

Figure 20.4 Labeled sagittal sonoanatomy for caudal block (sacrococcygeal ligament, sacral spine (SS), caudal space, anterior sacral foramina (ASF)).

dose saline is injected. Correct position of the needle in the caudal epidural space is confirmed by a localized turbulence or a dilation of the hiatus (displacing the sacrococcygeal ligament upward) during injection. The LA is injected slowly under ultrasound visualization. With transverse ultrasound scanning, the spread observed from the needle is rather wide and it may be difficult to ensure accurate location of the tip.

Table 20.1 Volume of local anesthetic (LA) in single shot caudal block (bupivacaine/levobupivacaine 0.175–0.25% or ropivacaine 0.2%)

Site of incision	Volume (ml/kg)
S1 (ankle, knee surgery)	0.50
L1 (hip surgery, hernia repair)	0.75
T10 (abdominal subumbilical surgery)	1.00

A successful block is defined as no motor or hemodynamic response (increase in mean arterial pressure or heart rate of more than 15% compared with baseline values) to skin incision and to subsequent surgical procedure.

A single shot caudal block provides relatively brief analgesia (4–8 h). Adjuvants are used to prolong the duration of analgesia. A dose of 33–50 µg/kg of preservative-free morphine in the caudal epidural solution improves the quality and duration of analgesia (12–24 h), but can be associated with itching, nausea, urinary retention, and respiratory depression. High doses (>33 µg/kg) require admission to a high dependency unit for respiratory monitoring (Krane et al., 1989).

The addition of clonidine (an α2-adrenergic agonist) 1–3 µg/kg, can provide prolonged analgesia (lasting for up to 12 h) without causing significant side effects. Doses greater than 2 µg/kg can be

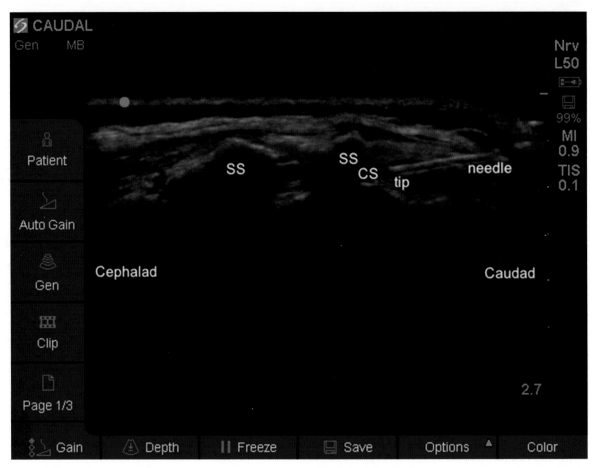

Figure 20.5 Ultrasound-guided caudal block with needle in situ. CS, caudal space; SS, sacral spine.

associated with increased sedation, bradycardia, hypotension, or respiratory depression. Clonidine should be avoided in young infants, as post-operative apnea can occur (Galante, 2005).

The addition of ketamine (a NMDA-receptor antagonist) to LA nearly triples the duration of analgesia. A dose of 0.5 mg/kg is considered safe (Semple et al., 1996). Preservative-free S-ketamine is available in some countries. Despite not being associated with significant side effects, there are still concerns regarding possible neurotoxicity (Vranken et al., 2006; Johr and Berger, 2012).

Technique failure is usually related to a suboptimal positioning of the probe or, in older patients, to increased sacrum ossification leading to inadequate view of the needle and anatomic landmarks.

Post-operative care

Quality of pain, motor power, and level of sensory block are assessed in the post-operative period according to hospital protocol (usually every 30 min). Care should be take to avoid contact with hot surfaces such as radiators. Bed rest for 2–3 hours is recommended with assisted mobilization to avoid pressure areas. The patient is monitored for possible complications: cardiovascular instability, respiratory depression (if caudal opioids used), nausea and vomiting, drowsiness, urinary retention, or prolonged motor blockade. A post-operative analgesia plan is very important in order to avoid severe pain after block resolution.

Clinical tips

- Successful performance of a caudal epidural starts with the accurate identification of the sacral hiatus.
- Placement of the probe at the level of coccyx with subsequent scanning toward the sacral canal will help the clinician to localize important landmarks.
- In infants and neonates, the ultrasound probe positioned in the sagittal plane allows an optimal visibility of sonoanatomy and LA spread.
- The needle is advanced at an angle of approximately 20 degrees with the skin so that it is parallel to the posterior surface of the sacrum.
- Visualize the spread of the LA within caudal epidural space or look for the anterior displacement of dura mater.
- Increased ossification of the spine, as child grows, can diminish the quality of the view on ultrasound.
- Adjuvants, such as clonidine (1–2 μg/kg), improve the duration and quality of analgesia with minimal side effects

Suggested reading

Brenner L, Marhofer P, Kettner SC, et al. (2011) Ultrasound assessment of cranial spread during caudal blockade in children: the effect of different volumes of local anaesthetics. *Br J Anaesth.* 107,229–35.

Dadure C, Raux O, Rochette A, Capdevila X. (2009) Interest of ultrasonographic guidance in paediatric regional anaesthesia. *Ann Fr Anesth Reanim.* 28(10), 878–84.

Ecoffey C, Lacroix F, Giaufré E, Orliaguet G, Courrèges P; Association des Anesthésistes Réanimateurs Pédiatriques d'Expression Française (ADARPEF). (2010) Epidemiology and morbidity of regional anesthesia in children: a follow-up one-year prospective survey of the French-Language Society of Paediatric Anaesthesiologists (ADARPEF). *Paediatr Anaesth.* 20,1061–9.

Galante D. (2005) Preoperative apnea in a preterm infant after caudal block with ropivacaine and clonidine. *Paediatr Anaesth.* 15,708–9.

Galante D. (2008) Ultrasound needle guidance in neonatal and infant caudal anesthesia. *Paediatr Anaesth.* 18,1233–4.

Ghai B., Bala I., Bhardwaj N. (2005) Caudal block. *Paediatr Anaesth.* 15,900–6.

Ivani G. (2005) Caudal block: the 'no turn technique'. *Paediatr Anaesth.* 15,83–4.

Ivani G, Mosseti V. (2009) Pediatric regional anesthesia. *Minerva Anestesiol.* 75(10),577–83.

Johr M, Berger TM. Caudal blocks. (2012) *Paediatr Anaesth.* 22, 44–50.

Kim J, Shin S, Lee H, Kil HK. (2013) Tethered spinal cord syndrome detected during ultrasound for caudal block in a child with single urological anomaly. *Korean J Anesthesiol.* 64(6),552–3.

Krane EJ. (1988) Delayed respiratory depression in a child after caudal epidural morphine. *Anesth Analg.* 67,79–82.

Krane EJ, Tyler DC, Jacobson LE. (1989) The dose response of caudal morphine in children. *Anesthesiology.* 71,48–52.

Lee JJ, Rubin AP. (1994). Comparison of a bupivacaine-clonidine mixture with plain bupivacaine for caudal analgesia in children. *Br J Anaesth.* 72,258–62.

Park JH, Koo BN, Kim JY, et al. (2006) Determination of the optimal angle for needle insertion during caudal block in children using ultrasound imaging. *Anaesthesia.* 61,946–9.

Polaner DM, Taenzer AH, Walker BJ, et al. (2012) Pediatric Regional Anesthesia Network (PRAN): a multi-institutional study of the use and incidence of complications of pediatric regional anesthesia. *Anest Analg.* 115(6),1353–64.

Raghunathan K, Schwartz D, Connelly NR. (2008) Determining the accuracy of caudal needle placement in children: a comparison of the swoosh test and ultrasonography. *Paediatr Anaesth.* 18,606–12.

Roberts S, Galvez I. (2005) Ultrasound assessment of caudal catheter position in infants. *Paediatr Anaesth.* 15,429–32.

Roberts S, Guruswamy V, Galvez I. (2005) Caudal injectate can be reliably imaged using portable ultrasound – a preliminary study. *Paediatr Anaesth.* 15, 948–52.

Schwartz D, Dunn SM, Connelly NR. (2006) Ultrasound and caudal blocks in children. *Paediatr Anaesth.* 16,900–1.

Schwartz D, Raghunathan K, Dunn S et al. (2008) Ultrasonography and pediatric caudals. *Anesth Analg.* 106,97–9.

Semple D, Findlow D, Aldridge LM, Doyle E. (1996) The optimal dose of ketamine for caudal epidural blockade in children. *Anaesthesia.* 51(12),1170–2.

Shin SK, Hong JY, Kim WO et al. (2009) Ultrasound evaluation of the sacral area and comparison of sacral interspinous and hiatal approach for caudal block in children. *Anesthesiology.* 111,1135–40.

Silvani P, Camporesi A, Agostino MR, Salvo I. (2006) Caudal anesthesia in pediatrics: an update. *Minerva Anestesiol.* 72(6),453–9.

Vranken JH, Troost D, de Haan P et al. (2006) Severe toxic damage to the rabbit spinal cord after intrathecal administration of preservative-free S[+]-ketamine. *Anesthesiology.* 105,813–18.

Wang L., Hu X., Zhang Y, Chang X. (2013) A randomized comparison of caudal block by sacral hiatus injection under ultrasound guidance with traditional sacral canal injection in children. *Paediatr Anaesth.* 23,395–400.

21

Ultrasound-guided facial blocks

Chrystelle Sola and Christophe Dadure

Clinical use

Useful regional anesthesia can be applied for both acute and chronic pain management either as a diagnostic or therapeutic procedure of the face (Han et al., 2008). Resection of skin lesions, face lacerations, nose fracture or surgery, and cleft lip repair are the most common surgical pediatric procedures suitable for regional anesthesia (Dadure et al. 2012; Suresh and Voronov, 2012). As a result of the close vicinity of the cranial and cervical nerves to many vital structures in a compact area, the efficacy and safety of cephalic blocks are based on optimal knowledge of the neighboring anatomic relationships of the selected nerve, its deep and superficial courses, and the final sensory territory. Rare, severe complications are reported during the performance of these blocks; however, as with other regional anesthesia techniques, hematoma formation, persistent paresthesia, intravascular injection, and organ lesions are still possible. Nerve damage by compression remains the main risk after

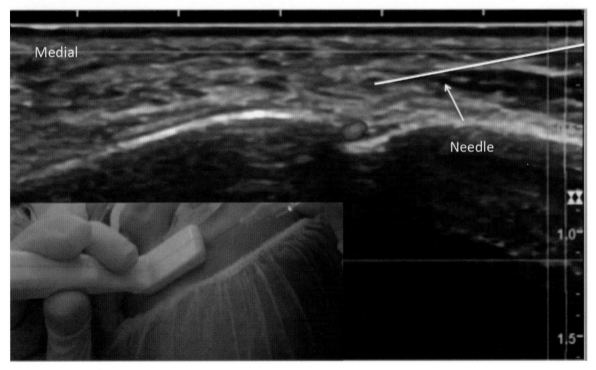

Figure 21.1 Probe placement and puncture site location for supraorbital nerve block. Ultrasound transverse view of disruption of the bone table at the foramina and vessel identification using color Doppler.

Ultrasound-Guided Regional Anesthesia in Children, ed. Mannion et al. Published by Cambridge University Press.
© Cambridge University Press 2015.

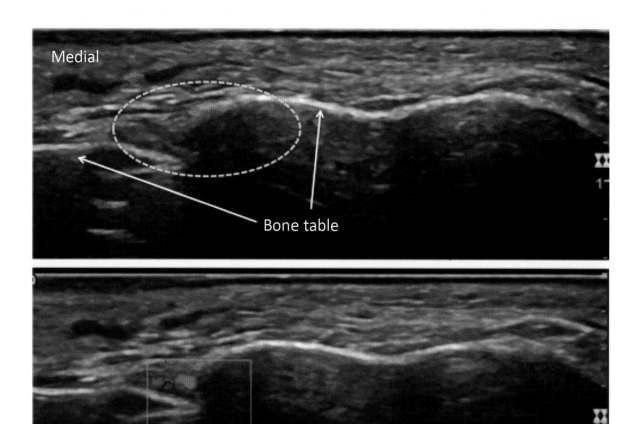

Medial

Bone table

Figure 21.2 The infraorbital nerve block: ultrasound transverse view of disruption of the bone table (broken yellow circle) at the foramina and vessels identification using color Doppler.

anatomic landmark superficial trigeminal nerves blocks (see below). With these concerns, ultrasound-guided techniques, because of the ability to visualize the anatomic structures and local anesthetic (LA) injection, provide for improved and possibly safer facial blocks.

Clinical sonoanatomy and landmarks

All sensory innervation of the face is dependent on the trigeminal nerve (fifth or V cranial nerve) associated with the C2–C4 cervical nerve roots that constitute the superficial cervical plexus. Facial peripheral nerve blocks are divided into two categories: superficial trigeminal nerve blocks and deeper blocks such as the suprazygomatic maxillary block.

Superficial trigeminal nerve blocks

For superficial trigeminal nerve blocks, the LA solution should be injected in close proximity to the three individual terminal superficial branches of the trigeminal nerve divisions: frontal nerve (from the ophthalmic nerve, V1 division); infraorbital nerve (from the maxillary nerve, V2 division); and mental nerve (sensory terminal branch of the mandibular nerve, V3 division), which supply innervation to the front half of the head, face, mouth, tongue, and chin. Each nerve is located close to the foramen by which it emerges and that is usually on a vertical line centered through the pupil. Ultrasound imaging to detect the foramen for each superficial trigeminal nerve block was first described as an easy and safe method (Tsui, 2009). Using a high frequency linear transducer, the bone table appears as a hyperechoic linear edge (white line) with an underlying

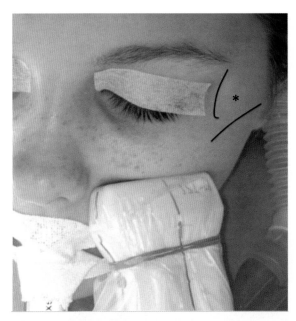

Figure 21.3 The suprazygomatic maxillary nerve block: probe placement and puncture site location (*) at the angle formed inferiorly by the superior edge of the zygomatic arch and anteriorly by the posterior margin of the lateral orbital rim.

anechoic (dark) shadow. At the foramina of these three nerves, disruption within the hyperechoic line indicates a discontinuity in the bone (a "bone gap" or "disruption of the bone table" concept) (Figures 21.1 and 21.2). In addition, ultrasound can visualize satellite vessels close to each nerve using color Doppler. The real-time view of LA spread can avoid intravascular injection, and the risk of nerve injury by compression after accidental injection into the foramen.

The probe is located transversally above the orbital rim to localize the supraorbital foramen (frontal nerve). The infraorbital foramen image can be achieved by positioning the ultrasound probe horizontally or vertically in the sagittal plane (infraorbital nerve). Slight translation movements from medial to lateral along the lower orbital margin are performed to highlight the disruption of the bone table. Finally, the mental foramen is localized using a transverse or sagittal plane with dynamic scanning between the upper and lower borders of the mandible at the level of the second inferior premolar with scanning in the cephalic direction (mental nerve).

Suprazygomatic maxillary block

The maxillary nerve (V2 – second division of the trigeminal nerve) exits the skull through the

rotundum foramen. The majority of its terminal branches (zygomatic branches, superior alveolar nerve, pterygopalatine and parasympathetic branches, palatine and pharyngeal branches) arise in the pterygopalatine fossa to supply sensory innervation of the cutaneous temporo-zygomatic area, the lower eyelid, the nasal septum, and of the lateral nasal wall, upper lip and teeth, the soft and bone palates, and maxillary sinus. At the upper part of the pterygopalatine fossa, the maxillary nerve is accessible for a complete maxillary block. In children, the ultrasound-guided suprazygomatic approach of maxillary nerve in pterygopalatine fossa seems to be safe and easily reproducible (Sola et al., 2012). The high frequency probe is placed in the infrazygomatic area, over the maxilla, with an inclination of 45 degrees in both the frontal and horizontal planes (Figure 21.3). The probe location allows visualization of the pterygopalatine fossa, limited anteriorly by the maxilla and posteriorly by the greater wing of the sphenoid (Figure 21.4). The needle is advanced using the out-of-plane approach. Real-time ultrasound guidance allows direct localization of the internal maxillary artery, needle-tip positioning –which is easily identified by movements applied to the needle and the spread of LA solution within the pterygopalatine fossa.

Block performance
Superficial trigeminal nerve blocks

The superficial trigeminal nerve blocks are usually performed with the patient in the supine position and the head in neutral position. Performing these blocks is preceded by a subcutaneous injection of a small volume of LA close to the emergence of the three terminal branches of their respective foramen. Fine and short needles (25–30-gauge, 25 mm) and small syringes (1–5 ml) will be suitable for these blocks. For surgical anesthesia, 0.1 mL/kg to a maximum of 5 ml of LA may be used, while diagnostic or therapeutic volumes will be much smaller (0.5–1.0 mL). Position the probe in a transverse plane at the level of each foramen – subtle translation movements help to identify the hypoechoic disruption of the bone table indicating the foramen. After the verification of each orifice using color Doppler, an in-plane approach can be easily employed in order to ensure safe injection, close to but outside the foramen. Once the block is performed, gentle pressure is applied for better LA spread and to prevent ecchymosis or hematoma formation.

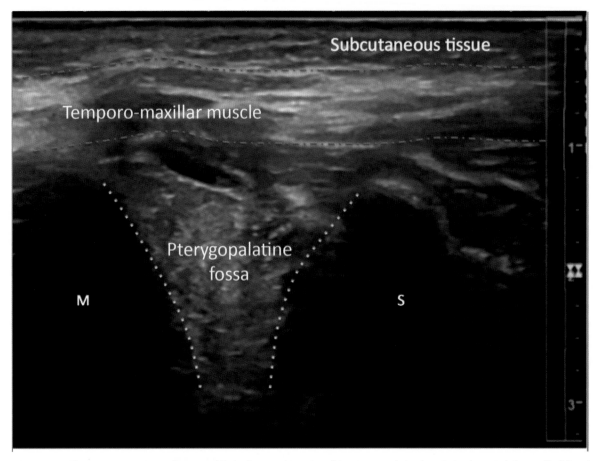

Figure 21.4 The suprazygomatic maxillary nerve block: ultrasound imaging of the pterygopalatine fossa limited anteriorly by maxilla (M) and posteriorly by the greater wing of the sphenoid (S).

Suprazygomatic maxillary block

The suprazygomatic maxillary nerve block is performed using a 25-gauge 50 mm needle according to the following conventional anatomical landmarks: the patient is supine with the head in neutral position or turned slightly to the opposite side. The needle entry point is situated at the angle formed inferiorly by the superior edge of the zygomatic arch and anteriorly by the posterior margin of the lateral orbital rim (Figure 21.3). The needle is inserted perpendicular to the skin and advanced to reach the greater wing of the sphenoid at approximately 10–15 mm depth. The needle is then reoriented in a caudal and posterior direction and advanced 35–45 mm deep to the pterygopalatine fossa (Figure 21.4) using the out-of-plane approach. With the probe positioned over the maxilla, in the infrazygomatic area, the needle tip is easily identified during movements. After a negative aspiration test for blood, 0.15–0.20 ml/kg (with a max. of 5 ml) of LA is slowly injected under direct visualization of the spread of the solution in the pterygopalatine fossa.

Clinical tips

- Ultrasound facial blocks described include the superficial trigeminal nerve blocks and the suprazygomatic maxillary block.
- Ultrasound facial blocks are indicated for post-operative analgesia after cleft lip repair, facial lacerations, nasal surgery, and chronic facial pain.
- Color Doppler is useful for identifying small blood vessels and, therefore, avoiding intravascular injection.

Suggested reading

Dadure C, Sola C, Choquet O, Capdevila X. (2012) Peripheral nerve blocks of the face in children. *Ann Fr Anesth Reanim.* 31, e17–20.

Han KR, Kim C, Chae YJ, Kim DW. (2008) Efficacy and safety of high concentration lidocaine for trigeminal nerve block in patients with trigeminal neuralgia. *Int J Clin Pract.* 62,248–54.

Sola C, Raux O, Savath L, et al. (2012) Ultrasound guidance characteristics and efficiency of suprazygomatic maxillary nerve blocks in infants: a descriptive prospective study. *Paediatr Anaesth.* 22,841–6.

Suresh S, Voronov P. (2012) Head and neck blocks in infants, children, and adolescents. *Paediatr Anaesth.* 22,81–7.

Tsui BC. (2009) Ultrasound imaging to localize foramina for superficial trigeminal nerve block. *Can J Anaesth.* 56,704–6.

Appendix: Muscle innervation, origin, insertion, and action

Table A.1 Superficial muscle group of the shoulder

Name	Innervation and specific nerve root	Origin	Insertion	Action
Trapezius	Accessory nerve (CN XI), C3, C4	External occipital protuberance, nuchal ligament, medial superior nuchal line, spinous processes of C7–T12	Posterior border of the lateral third of clavicle, acromion process and spine of scapula	Rotation, retraction, elevation, and depression of scapula.
Deltoid	Axillary nerve (C5, C6)	Anterior border and upper surface of lateral third of clavicle, acromion, and scapular spine	Deltoid tuberosity of the humerus	Abduction, flexion, and extension of the shoulder
Levator scapulae	C3, C4, C5	Transverse process of C1 and C2, posterior tubercles of transverse process of C3 and C4	Posteromedial border of scapula	Elevates the scapula
Rhomboid major	Dorsal scapular nerve (C4, C5)	Lower aspect of ligamentum nuchae, spinous processes of C7 and T1	Posteromedial border of scapula	Elevates and retracts the scapula
Rhomboid minor	Dorsal scapular nerve (C4, C5)	Spinous processes of T2–T5 and associated supraspinous ligament	Posteromedial border of scapula	Elevates and retracts the scapula

Table A.2 Deep muscle group of the shoulder

Name	Innervation and specific nerve root	Origin	Insertion	Action
Supraspinatus	Suprascapular nerve (C5, C6)	Medial two-thirds of supraspinous fossa of scapula	Greater tubercle of humerus	Initiates abduction of arm at shoulder
Infraspinatus	Suprascapular nerve (C5, C6)	Medial two-thirds of infraspinous fossa of scapula	Greater tubercle of humerus	Lateral rotation of arm at shoulder
Teres major	Inferior subscapular nerve (C5, C6, C7)	Posterior surface of inferior angle of scapula	Intertubercular sulcus of anterior surface of humerus	Medial rotation and extension of shoulder
Teres minor	Axillary nerve (C5, C6)	Upper two-thirds of posterior surface of scapula	Greater tubercle of humerus	Lateral rotation of arm at shoulder
Long head of Triceps brachii	Axillary nerve (C5, C6)	Infraglenoid tubercle	Olecranon process of ulna	Accessory abductor of shoulder

Ultrasound-Guided Regional Anesthesia in Children, ed. Mannion et al. Published by Cambridge University Press.
© Cambridge University Press 2015.

Table A.3 Anterior and posterior muscles of the arm

Name	Innervation and specific nerve root	Origin	Insertion	Action
Coracobrachialis	Musculocutaneous nerve (C5, C6, C7)	Apex of coracoid process	Medial aspect of humerus	Flexes the arm at the shoulder
Brachialis	Musculocutaneous nerve (C5, C6, C7)	Anterior aspect of humerus	Tuberosity of ulna	Flexes forearm at elbow
Biceps brachii	Musculocutaneous nerve (C5, C6, C7)	Long head: supraglenoid tubercle of scapula. Short head: apex of coracoid process	Tuberosity of radius	Flexes and supinates forearm at elbow
Triceps brachii	Axillary nerve (C5, C6), radial nerve (C6, C7, C8)	Long head: infraglenoid tubercle of scapula. Medial head: posterior surface of humerus. Lateral head: posterior surface of humerus	Olecranon process	Extends forearm at elbow, long head extends and adducts shoulder

Table A.4 Superficial muscle group of the gluteal region

Name	Innervation and specific nerve root	Origin	Insertion	Action
Gluteus maximus	Inferior gluteal nerve (L4, L5, S1, S2)	Gluteal surface of ilium, posterior surface of sacrum, sacrotuberous ligament, superior aspect of coccyx	Superior aspect of iliotibial band, gluteal tuberosity of femur	Extension, external rotation, and abduction of the hip joint Stabilizes knee via tightening of iliotibial band
Gluteus medius	Superior gluteal nerve (L4, L5, S1)	Gluteal surface of ilium between anterior and posterior gluteal line	Tip and lateral margin of greater trochanter (anteriorly and posteriorly)	Abduction of the hip joint. Internal and external rotation of the hip joint
Gluteus minimus	Superior gluteal nerve (L4, L5, S1)	Gluteal surface of ilium between anterior and inferior gluteal line	Tip and lateral margin of greater trochanter (anteriorly and posteriorly)	Abduction of the hip joint. Internal and external rotation of the hip joint
Tensor fasciae latae	Superior gluteal nerve (L4, L5, S1)	Lateral aspect of iliac crest	Iliotibial band	Knee stabilization during flexion

Table A.5 Deep muscle group of the gluteal region

Name	Innervation and specific nerve root	Origin	Insertion	Action
Piriformis	Nerve to piriformis (L5, S1)	Sacral segments 3–5, superior border of greater sciatic notch	Inner surface of greater trochanter	External rotation, abduction and extension of the hip joint
Obturator internus	Nerve to obturator internus (L5, S1, S2)	Medial surface of the obturator membrane	Trochanteric fossa	Extension and adduction of the hip joint, external rotation of the hip
Gemellus superior	Nerve to obturator internus (L5, S1, S2)	Ischial spine	Trochanteric fossa	
Gemellus inferior	Nerve to obturator internus (L5, S1, S2)	Ischial tuberosity	Trochanteric fossa	
Quadratus femoris	Nerve to quadratus femoris (L4, L5, S1)	Ischial tuberosity (lateral border)	Intertrochanteric crest	Adduction and external rotation of the hip

Table A.6 Muscles originating from the abdominal wall and acting on the hip

Name	Innervation and specific nerve root	Origin	Insertion	Action
Psoas	L2, L3	Vertebral bodies of T12, L1, L2, L3, L4, L5	Lesser trochanter, medial aspect of linea aspera	Lateral flexion and extension of the vertebral column, flexion and internal rotation of the hip joint
Iliacus	L2, L3	Iliac fossa, anterior inferior iliac spine (AIIS)	Lesser trochanter, medial aspect of linea aspera	Lateral flexion and extension of the vertebral column, flexion and internal rotation of the hip joint

Table A.7 Anterior muscle group of the thigh

Name	Innervation and specific nerve root	Origin	Insertion	Action
Rectus femoris (straight head) Rectus femoris (reflected head)	Nerve to rectus femoris (L2, L3, L4)	Anterior inferior iliac spine (ASIS) Superior border of acetabulum	Patella ligament, upper border of patella	Flexion of the hip joint. Extension of the knee joint
Vastus medialis	Nerve to vastus medialis (L2, L3, L4)	Lower section of intertrochanteric line, medial aspect of linea aspera, medial epicondylar line	Patella ligament, upper border of patella	Extension of the knee joint
Vastus intermedialis	Nerve to vastus intermedialis (L2, L3)	Upper section of anterior and lateral surface of femur	Patella ligament, upper border of patella	
Vastus lateralis	Nerve to vastus lateralis (L2, L3, L4)	Upper section of intertrochanteric line, greater trochanter, lower margin of linea aspera, lateral epicondylar line	Patella ligament, upper border of patella	
Sartorius	Femoral nerve (L2, L3)	ASIS	Medial aspect of tibial tuberosity	Flexion, external rotation and abduction of hip joint. Flexion and internal rotation of the knee joint

Table A.8 Medial muscle group of the thigh

Name	Innervation and specific nerve root	Origin	Insertion	Action
Obturator externus	Obturator nerve (L2, L3, L4)	Lower lateral surface of obturator membrane, inferior pubic ramus	Trochanteric fossa	Adduction and external rotation of the hip joint
Pectineus	Femoral nerve (L2, L3), sometimes obturator nerve (L2, L3, L4)	Body of the pubis	Pectineal line of femur	Adduction, external rotation and flexion of the hip joint
Gracilis	Obturator nerve (L2, L3, L4)	Medial aspect of inferior pubic ramus	Medial aspect of the tibial tuberosity	Adduction, external rotation and flexion of the hip joint. Flexion and internal rotation of the knee joint
Adductor brevis	Obturator nerve (L2, L3, L4)	Inferior pubic ramus	Upper third of linea aspera	Adduction, external rotation and flexion of the hip joint
Adductor longus	Anterior division of obturator nerve (L2, L3)	Pubic crest	Medial third of linea aspera	Adduction, external rotation and flexion of the hip joint
Adductor magnus	Posterior division of obturator nerve (L3, L4). Tibial portion of sciatic nerve	Inferior pubic ramus, ischial tuberosity	Lower half of linea aspera, adductor tubercle	Adduction and external rotation of the hip joint. Can also contribute to flexion and extension of the hip joint

Table A.9 Posterior muscle group of the thigh

Name	Innervation and specific nerve root	Origin	Insertion	Action
Biceps femoris	Sciatic nerve (L4, L5, S1, S2)	*Long head:* Ischial tuberosity *Short head:* Middle third of linea aspera	Head of the fibula, covering lateral collateral ligament	Extension, adduction and external rotation of the hip joint Flexion and external rotation of the knee joint
Semimembranosus	Sciatic nerve (L4, L5, S1)	Ischial tuberosity	Posterior to the medial condyle of the tibia	Extension, adduction, and internal rotation of the hip joint Flexion and internal rotation of the knee joint
Semitendinosus	Sciatic nerve (L4, L5, S1)	Ischial tuberosity	Medial surface of the tibial tuberosity	Extension, adduction, and internal rotation of the hip joint Flexion and external rotation of the knee joint

Index

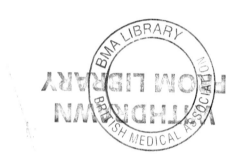